T0226541

Innovations in Foot and Ankle Surgery

Editor

GUIDO A. LAPORTA

CLINICS IN PODIATRIC MEDICINE AND SURGERY

www.podiatric.theclinics.com

Consulting Editor
THOMAS J. CHANG

October 2018 • Volume 35 • Number 4

ELSEVIER

1600 John F. Kennedy Boulevard • Suite 1800 • Philadelphia, Pennsylvania, 19103-2899

http://www.theclinics.com

CLINICS IN PODIATRIC MEDICINE AND SURGERY Volume 35, Number 4
October 2018 ISSN 0891-8422, ISBN-13: 978-0-323-64116-6

Editor: Lauren Boyle
Developmental Editor: Sara Watkins

Clinics in Podiatric Medicine and Surgery (ISSN 0891-8422) is published quarterly by Elsevier Inc., 360 Park Avenue South, New York, NY 10010-1710. Months of issue are January, April, July, and October. Business and Editorial Offices: 1600 John F. Kennedy Blvd., Ste. 1800, Philadelphia, PA 19103-2899. Customer Service Office: 3251 Riverport Lane, Maryland Heights, MO 63043. Periodicals postage paid at New York, NY and additional mailing offices. Subscription prices are $294.00 per year for US individuals, $544.00 per year for US institutions, $100.00 per year for US students and residents, $382.00 per year for Canadian individuals, $657.00 for Canadian institutions, $439.00 for international individuals, $657.00 per year for international institutions and $220.00 per year for Canadian and foreign students/residents. To receive student/resident rate, orders must be accompanied by name of affiliated institution, date of term, and the *signature* of program/residency coordinator on institution letterhead. Orders will be billed at individual rate until proof of status is received. Foreign air speed delivery is included in all *Clinics* subscription prices. All prices are subject to change without notice. POSTMASTER: Send address changes to *Clinics in Podiatric Medicine and Surgery*, Elsevier Health Sciences Division, Subscription Customer Service, 3251 Riverport Lane, Maryland Heights, MO 63043. **Customer Service: 1-800-654-2452 (US). From outside of the US, call 314-447-8871. Fax: 314-447-8029. E-mail: JournalsCustomerService-usa@elsevier.com (for print support); JournalsOnlineSupport-usa@elsevier. com (for online support).**

Reprints. For copies of 100 or more of articles in this publication, please contact the Commercial Reprints Department, Elsevier Inc., 360 Park Avenue South, New York, NY 10010-1710. Tel.: 212-633-3874; Fax: 212-633-3820; E-mail: reprints@elsevier.com.

Clinics in Podiatric Medicine and Surgery is covered in *MEDLINE/PubMed (Index Medicus)* and *EMBASE/Excerpta Medica*.

Contributors

CONSULTING EDITOR

THOMAS J. CHANG, DPM
Clinical Professor and Past Chairman, Department of Podiatric Surgery, California College of Podiatric Medicine, Faculty, The Podiatry Institute, Redwood Orthopedic Surgery Associates, Santa Rosa, California, USA

EDITOR

GUIDO A. LaPORTA, DPM, MS, FACFAS
Director, Podiatric Medical Education, Podiatric Residency Program, Geisinger Community Medical Center, Scranton, Pennsylvania, USA; Residency Program Director, Our Lady of Lourdes Memorial Hospital, Binghamton, New York, USA; Professor of Surgery, Geisinger Commonwealth Medical College, North Abington Township, Pennsylvania, USA; LaPorta and Associates PC, Dunmore, Pennsylvania, USA

AUTHORS

FRANZ BIRKHOLTS, MD
Walk A Mile Centre, Lyttelton, Pretoria, South Africa

ALEXANDER M. CHERKASHIN, MD
Assistant Professor, Department of Orthopedic Surgery, UT Southwestern Medical School, Texas Scottish Rite Hospital for Children, Dallas, Texas, USA

CRAIG E. CLIFFORD, DPM, MHA, FACFAS, FACFAOM
Franciscan Orthopedic Associates at St Francis, Federal Way, Washington, USA

ALISON D'ANDELET, DPM, MHA
Podiatric Medical Education, Our Lady of Lourdes Memorial Hospital, Binghamton, New York, USA

LEE M. HLAD, DPM, FACFAS
Fellowship Trained Foot and Ankle Surgeon, Private Practice, Faculty, Foot and Ankle Surgery, Residence, Grant Medical Center, Community Physician, Nationwide Children's Hospital, Columbus, Ohio, USA

BYRON HUTCHINSON, DPM, FACFAS
Franciscan Foot & Ankle Associates: Highline Clinic, Seattle, Washington, USA

ANDREAS C. KAIKIS, DPM
Resident, Department of Podiatric Surgery, University of Pennsylvania, Penn Presbyterian Medical Center, Philadelphia, Pennsylvania, USA

GUIDO A. LaPORTA, DPM, MS, FACFAS
Director, Podiatric Medical Education, Podiatric Residency Program, Geisinger
Community Medical Center, Scranton, Pennsylvania, USA; Residency Program Director,
Our Lady of Lourdes Memorial Hospital, Binghamton, New York, USA; Professor
of Surgery, Geisinger Commonwealth Medical College, North Abington Township,
Pennsylvania, USA; LaPorta and Associates PC, Dunmore, Pennsylvania, USA

KEVIN M. McCANN, DPM, MHA, FACFAS
St Cloud Orthopedics, Sartell, Minnesota, USA

LAUREN M. PELUCACCI, DPM
Resident Physician, Geisinger Community Medical Center, Scranton, Pennsylvania, USA

WILLIAM A. PIERCE, BS ENG
Texas Scottish Rite Hospital for Children, Dallas, Texas, USA

THOMAS M. ROCCHIO, DPM, FACFAS
PA Foot and Ankle Associates, Allentown, Pennsylvania, USA; Easton Hospital Wound
Healing Center, Easton, Pennsylvania, USA

ALI M. SALEH, DPM, BA
Resident, PGY-1, St. Mary's General Podiatric Residency, Passaic, New Jersey, USA

MIKHAIL L. SAMCHUKOV, MD
Associate Professor, Department of Orthopedic Surgery, UT Southwestern Medical
School, Texas Scottish Rite Hospital for Children, Dallas, Texas, USA

MARK SHEARER, DPM, ACFAS
Fellow, Northern New Jersey Reconstructive Foot and Ankle Fellowship, Lyndhurst,
New Jersey, USA; Residency Training, Our Lady of Lourdes Memorial Hospital,
Binghamton, New York, USA

HELEN SHNOL, DPM
Department of Graduate Medical Education and Podiatric Surgery, Our Lady of
Lourdes Memorial Hospital, Binghamton, New York, USA

NOMAN A. SIDDIQUI, DPM, MHA
International Center for Limb Lengthening, Rubin Institute for Advanced Orthopedics,
Sinai Hospital of Baltimore, Baltimore, Maryland, USA

PAUL A. STASKO, DPM, FACFAS
Podiatry-Foot and Ankle Surgery, Rochester Regional Health-Fingerlakes Bone and Joint
Center, Geneva, New York, USA

MICHAEL SUBIK, DPM, FACFAS
Director Podiatric Residency, St. Mary's General Hospital, Passaic, New Jersey, USA;
Founder and Director, The North Jersey Reconstructive Foot and Ankle Fellowship,
Lyndhurst, New Jersey, USA

JACOB WYNES, DPM, MS
Assistant Professor, Department of Orthopaedics, University of Maryland School of
Medicine, Baltimore, Maryland, USA

Contents

Foreword: Innovations in Foot and Ankle Surgery ix

Thomas J. Chang

Preface: Back to the Future xi

Guido A. LaPorta

Subchondroplasty: Treatment of Bone Marrow Lesions in the Lower Extremity 367

Lauren M. Pelucacci and Guido A. LaPorta

Bone marrow lesions are associated with pain, disease progression, and cartilage loss in inflammatory and noninflammatory conditions, and are related to mechanical loading and subchondral stress. Treatment, particularly in the foot and ankle, is challenging. In the subchondroplasty procedure, flowable, synthetic, calcium phosphate bone filler is injected into the defect region, improving subchondral bone integrity and allowing remodeling back into healthy cancellous bone. The procedure is a promising treatment option for bone marrow lesions, particularly in the foot and ankle. The benefits are a minimally invasive procedure with early return to weightbearing.

Resorbable Polymer Pin Inserted with Ultrasound Activated BoneWelding Technique Compared with a Screw for Osteotomy Fixation in the Reverse L Bunion Correction 373

Thomas M. Rocchio

Screw fixation of an osteotomy in the first metatarsal for bunion correction represents a compromise. The need to return to the operating room for removal exposes patients to added anesthesia risk, expense, time, and possible surgical complications. This article compares screw fixation with a novel new bioresorbable polymer pin that is inserted with an ultrasound activated BoneWelding technique to fixate a bunion correction using a reversed L osteotomy. This article reviews and discusses the present benefits of a time-tested osteotomy that, when fixated with this polymer and BoneWelding technique, offer new solutions for a compromised patient population.

Minimally Invasive Bunion Correction 387

Noman A. Siddiqui and Guido A. LaPorta

Hallux valgus is a common condition that results in lateral deviation of the hallux and medial deviation of the metatarsal. When conservative management fails, surgical management is often necessary. More than 150 procedures have been described, and most recommend an open approach. More recently, a minimally invasive approach to bunion correction has gained popularity among surgeons. The authors have been performing a minimally invasive percutaneous method of bunion correction with positive outcomes. This article presents case examples and a systematic approach for correction of this common foot condition.

3D Printed Total Talar Replacement: A Promising Treatment Option for Advanced Arthritis, Avascular Osteonecrosis, and Osteomyelitis of the Ankle   403

Helen Shnol and Guido A. LaPorta

Advanced ankle arthritis, avascular osteonecrosis, and osteomyelitis of the ankle remain a surgical challenge in the foot and ankle arena with limited treatment options. Multiple medical comorbidities contribute to total loss of the talus. Collapse of the talar body as a complication of total ankle arthroplasty, talectomy in infection, and septic talus necrosis or severe bone defects caused by tumor resection may result in need for total talar replacement. Ankle arthrodesis and tibiocalcaneal fusion after talectomy can produce severe disability of the ankle and foot. Total ankle replacement is a viable option for treatment of end-stage ankle arthritis in appropriate patient populations.

Treatment Strategies and Frame Configurations in the Management of Foot and Ankle Deformities   423

Alexander M. Cherkashin, Mikhail L. Samchukov, and Franz Birkholts

To provide standardized nomenclature for various hexapod frame configurations for foot and ankle deformity correction, a unique classification of the hexapod external fixators was proposed. This classification is based on number of correction levels, secured anatomic blocks, and direction of the strut attachment. It allows the combination of all different foot and ankle frame assemblies into a few standard hexapod configurations, irrespective of which external fixator is used.

Biomechanical Considerations in Foot and Ankle Circular External Fixation: Maintenance of Wire Tension   443

Mikhail L. Samchukov, Craig E. Clifford, Kevin M. McCann, Alexander M. Cherkashin, Byron Hutchinson, and William A. Pierce

Initial tensioning of the forefoot wires to 130 kg followed by simultaneous tensioning of the calcaneal wires to 90 kg and using the rigid double-row foot plate closed anteriorly via threaded rods produce maximum preservation of the initial wire tension during foot circular external fixation.

Essentials of Deformity Planning   457

Paul A. Stasko and Lee M. Hlad

Learning the essentials of deformity planning is the basis for the treatment of simple and complex deformities. Understanding the planes of deformity, radiographic correlation, and clinical correlations allows the surgeon to treat the condition with deeper knowledge of deformity, leading to improved deformity correction.

Current Advancements in Ankle Arthrodiastasis   467

Jacob Wynes and Andreas C. Kaikis

Ankle arthrodiastasis offers an option for patients with end-stage primary or posttraumatic ankle osteoarthritis. The process allows for a joint salvage procedure as an alternative to arthrodesis or ankle implant arthroplasty. The distraction within the joint optimizes the intraarticular environment to permit equilibration of hydrostatic pressure, promoting subchondral morphoangiogenesis, and decreases subchondral sclerosis, thereby mitigating pain. This article highlights new advances and useful adjunctive procedures in this interesting approach to the management of ankle pain secondary to loss of functional joint surface.

The Gradual and Acute Correction of Equinus Using External Fixation   481

Michael Subik, Mark Shearer, Ali M. Saleh, and Guido A. LaPorta

Equinus is one of the most common deformities noted in foot and ankle biomechanics that, at times, if not identified and managed properly, may lead to significant lower extremity pathology. With that being said, this deformity is also one that may be both underdiagnosed and undertreated. Treatment for equinus can range from conservative therapy to more aggressive surgical therapy. The purpose of this article is to review the clinical workup to properly identify the deformity and to explore the various treatment options for its timely management, which include gradual or acute correction of equinus using external fixation.

Lengthen, Alignment, and Beam Technique for Midfoot Charcot Neuroarthropathy   497

Guido A. LaPorta and Alison D'Andelet

Charcot neuroarthropathy is a disabling pathology in the foot and ankle. Midfoot Charcot is most common and results in progressive deformity. We describe a 2-step approach to surgical reconstruction, referred to as the lengthen, alignment, and beam technique. There is an initial surgery involving acute equinus correction through Achilles tendon lengthening and gradual correction with hexapod external fixation to align the deformity, followed by minimally invasive medial and lateral column beaming. This surgical protocol allows for adequate reduction of deformity. The second stage allows for rigid intramedullary fixation extending beyond the pathologic joints via a minimally invasive technique.

Midfoot Charcot Reconstruction   509

Noman A. Siddiqui and Guido A. LaPorta

Midfoot Charcot joints are complex problems that are most commonly seen in patients with peripheral neuropathy secondary to diabetes. The goal of management is to prevent pedal collapse, which can lead to ulceration, infection, and in some cases, amputation. Principles of surgical management should be centered on respecting the soft tissue, obtaining correction, maintaining correction, and supplementing with orthobiologics to achieve healing. The authors present strategies, case examples, and tips and tricks to treat this complex condition with external and internal fixation.

CLINICS IN PODIATRIC MEDICINE AND SURGERY

FORTHCOMING ISSUES

January 2019
Perioperative Considerations in the Surgical Patient
Jeffrey Shook, *Editor*

April 2019
Current Perspectives on Management of Calcaneal Fractures
Thomas S. Roukis, *Editor*

July 2019
Diabetes
Paul J. Kim, *Editor*

RECENT ISSUES

July 2018
Use of Biologics for Foot and Ankle Surgery
Adam S. Landsman, *Editor*

April 2018
Advanced Techniques in the Management of Foot and Ankle Trauma
Justin J. Fleming, *Editor*

January 2018
New Technologies in Foot and Ankle Surgery
Stephen A. Brigido, *Editor*

ISSUE OF RELATED INTEREST

Foot and Ankle Clinics, June 2017 (Vol. 22, No. 2)
Current Updates in Total Ankle Arthroplasty
J. Chris Coetzee, *Editor*
Available at: http://www.foot.theclinics.com/

Foreword

Innovations in Foot and Ankle Surgery

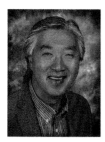

Thomas J. Chang, DPM
Consulting Editor

This issue of *Clinics in Podiatric Medicine and Surgery* is edited by Dr Guido LaPorta. Although Dr LaPorta has been in practice for over 45 years, he is continuously challenging accepted principles and techniques by finding improved surgical solutions to both routine and difficult problems. He is respected internationally as a gifted writer and educator, and even more importantly, he remains a student who listens eagerly and genuinely to anyone sharing their thoughts and experiences. I have observed this time and time again. He is a mentor to hundreds of foot and ankle surgeons, and he is a mentor of mine.

This issue brings a mix of simple and advanced topics. I know you will enjoy the variety of New Innovations topics. One article especially intrigued me, on "Minimally Invasive Bunion Correction". After doing bunion surgery for over 40 years, Dr LaPorta once again challenges himself and us to remain objective and always be open to consider other perspectives. I am grateful that he has assembled a team of experienced authors, all of whom have spent hours of time sharing their ideas with us. It is a privilege to have Dr LaPorta on this issue.

Regards,

Thomas J. Chang, DPM
Department of Podiatric Surgery
California College of Podiatric Medicine
The Podiatry Institute
Redwood Orthopedic Surgery Associates
208 Concourse Boulevard
Santa Rosa, CA 95403, USA

E-mail address:
thomaschang14@comcast.net

Clin Podiatr Med Surg 35 (2018) ix
https://doi.org/10.1016/j.cpm.2018.07.002
0891-8422/18/© 2018 Published by Elsevier Inc.

podiatric.theclinics.com

Preface

Back to the Future

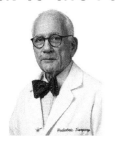

Guido A. LaPorta, DPM, MS, FACFAS
Editor

It has been an honor and a pleasure for me to be the Guest Editor for this issue of *Clinics in Podiatric Medicine and Surgery*. The field of foot and ankle surgery has seen many advances in the last twenty years, allowing the musculoskeletal surgeon to offer treatment options that were not available when I was in training. These advances may involve new treatment paradigms or, in some cases, improvements in established surgical techniques. These advancements have one thing in common: they benefit the patient. It has been an educational renaissance for me to be associated with these very talented colleagues.

I have been fortunate to be mentored by many great physicians, surgeons, and educators. I would like to acknowledge Drs Josh Gerbert, Lowell Weil Sr, James Ganley, and E. Dalton McGlamary for laying the foundation. I would also like to acknowledge Drs Dror Paley, John Herzenberg, and Charles Taylor, who recognized my interest in external fixation and did not hesitate to provide the opportunity for me to improve my skills. Last, I would like to thank Dr George Vito for taking the time and expending the effort to share his vast knowledge of the Ilizarov technique and its application to foot and ankle deformity with me.

I would like to dedicate this issue of the *Clinics in Podiatric Medicine and Surgery* to my former and future residents, students, and fellows, all of whom continue to inspire me to explore and improve my knowledge and skills.

Guido A. LaPorta, DPM, MS, FACFAS
Geisinger Community Medical Center
1800 Mulberry Street
Scranton, PA 18510, USA

Our Lady of Lourdes Memorial Hospital
169 Riverside Drive
Binghamton, NY 13905, USA

Geisinger Commonwealth Medical College
525 Pine Street
Scranton, PA 18510, USA

E-mail address:
glaporta@msn.com

Clin Podiatr Med Surg 35 (2018) xi
https://doi.org/10.1016/j.cpm.2018.07.001
0891-8422/18/© 2018 Published by Elsevier Inc.

Subchondroplasty

Treatment of Bone Marrow Lesions in the Lower Extremity

Lauren M. Pelucacci, DPM[a],*, Guido A. LaPorta, DPM, MS[a,b]

KEYWORDS

- Subchondroplasty • Bone marrow edema • Bone marrow lesions • Foot and ankle

KEY POINTS

- Bone marrow lesions of the foot and ankle are challenging to treat.
- Bone marrow lesions of the foot and ankle are associated with pain, limitation of function, and cartilage loss.
- Early diagnosis and treatment of bone marrow lesions are paramount to favorable patient outcomes.
- The subchondroplasty procedure is a novel, minimally invasive technique used to treat chronic nonhealing bone marrow lesions.
- The subchondroplasty procedure is a promising treatment option for bone marrow lesions of the foot and ankle.

A bone marrow lesion (BML), originally named regional migratory osteoporosis, is a clinical syndrome characterized by pain and reduced bone density on hip radiographs in the third trimester of pregnancy.[1] It was initially described in 1959 by Curtiss and Kincaid.[2] Since then, various terminology has been used to describe this clinical finding, such as transient osteoporosis of the hip, regional migratory osteoporosis, and reflex sympathetic dystrophy.

The term bone marrow edema (BME) was proposed by Hofmann and colleagues[3] in 2008 as a general term based on common MRI findings. Regardless of cause, BME presents as a nonspecific area of low signal intensity on T1-weighted MRI and intermediate or high signal intensity on T2-weighted MRI.[4]

Disclosure Statement: No disclosures.
^a Geisinger Community Medical Center, 1800 Mulberry Street, Scranton, PA 18510, USA;
^b LaPorta and Associates PC, 414 East Drinker Street, Dunmore, PA 18512, USA
* Corresponding author.
E-mail address: lmpelucacci@geisinger.edu

Clin Podiatr Med Surg 35 (2018) 367–371
https://doi.org/10.1016/j.cpm.2018.06.001   **podiatric.theclinics.com**
0891-8422/18/© 2018 Elsevier Inc. All rights reserved.

The cause underlying BME remains largely unknown. Recent histologic analysis of these lesions show an absence of edematous changes in many of these cases, which led to the adoption of the term BML.[5] Histologically, the lesions are characterized by fibrosis, lymphocytic infiltrates and increased vascularization. It is likely this increased vascularization is responsible for the water signal on MRI. BMLs have been associated with a variety of inflammatory and noninflammatory conditions, including trauma, osteoarthritis, inflammatory arthropathies, ischemia, infection, metabolic disorders, and neoplasms. In both inflammatory and noninflammatory conditions, the presence of BMLs is usually associated with pain, progression of disease, and cartilage loss.[6]

The presence of BMLs has been related to mechanical loading and increased subchondral stress, particularly in the hip, knee, ankle, and foot.[6] In 2001, Felson and colleagues[7,8] became the first to correlate BML with pain and subsequent osteoarthritis in the knee. In the MRI study, 77.5% of subjects with knee pain had BMLs deep to the subchondral bone.

Treatment of osteochondral lesions of the foot and ankle has proven to be challenging. For osteochondritis dissecans lesions of the talus, the standard of treatment has been arthroscopic interventions, which include retrograde drilling, bone marrow stimulation, and osteochondral autograft transportation. More recent techniques include cartilage autografts, such as autologous chondrocyte implantation, matrix-associated autologous chondrocyte implantation, and allograft tissues such as juvenile allograft cartilage.[9–12]

The subchondroplasty (SCP) procedure, developed in 2007, is a minimally invasive technique that uses an orthobiologic to treat chronic nonhealing BMLs. It is performed by injecting a flowable, synthetic, nanocrystalline calcium phosphate (CaP) bone filler into the region of the BML defect, using fluoroscopy as a guide.[13] When the CaP is injected, an endothermic reaction crystallizes the CaP to mimic the properties of healthy cancellous bone. This technique allows the CaP to be injected between subchondral cancellous trabeculae without damaging the existing bone scaffold.[14] SCP can be performed in conjunction with arthroscopy to improve accuracy of the desired injection location and to correct any intraarticular pathologic conditions. The goal of this procedure is to improve the integrity of the damaged subchondral bone and allow for remodeling back into healthy cancellous bone.[13]

Not many studies of the efficacy of SCP have been performed, particularly in the foot and ankle. Most of the literature has been in regard to the knee. Sharkey and Cohen[13] reported pain improvement in visual analog scale (VAS) scores by 4.3 points in 50 out of 57 subjects at 6-month follow-up of SCP of the knee. Bonadio and colleagues[14] performed SCP in 5 cases in the distal medial femoral condyle and the medial tibial plateau, all of which had VAS assessment drop from a mean of 7.8 preoperatively to a mean of 2.2 postoperatively at 24 weeks after surgery. Miller and Dunn[15] performed SCP of the ankle joint on 2 subjects, who both admit to having minimal pain of the ankle 10 months after surgery.

Though SCP has been primarily described in the lower extremity as being performed in the knee and talus, it can essentially be performed in any osseous structure of the foot with a symptomatic BML. In the authors' practices, SCP has been successfully performed in osseous structures of the rearfoot, midtarsus, and lesser tarsus.

Preoperatively, the patient presents with localized pain that has been unresponsive to conservative therapy, including offloading and short courses of antiinflammatory drug therapy. An MRI is obtained, which confirms or denies the presence of a BML, shows the specific location of the BML if it is present, and rules out any additional pathologic condition (**Fig. 1**).

The surgical technique for SCP of the foot is performed in a similar fashion to other osseous structures of the body. Fluoroscopy is used to identify the desired bone of the foot. A trocar and cannula are then inserted under fluoroscopic guidance, and approximately 0.5 to 1.5 mL of flowable CaP bone filler is injected directly into the BML (**Fig. 2**).

Immediately postoperatively, the patients are weightbearing as tolerated in a flat surgical shoe and generally notice an improvement in preoperative BML pain as early as 1 week following surgery.

The limited studies performed suggest that SCP may be a promising treatment option for BMLs, particularly in the foot and ankle. SCP offers the benefit of a minimally invasive procedure with early return to weightbearing, while restoring pathologic subchondral bone to healthy cancellous bone. It is hypothesized that improving the integrity of subchondral bone will result in a reduction of pain and progression of osteoarthritis in the lower extremity.

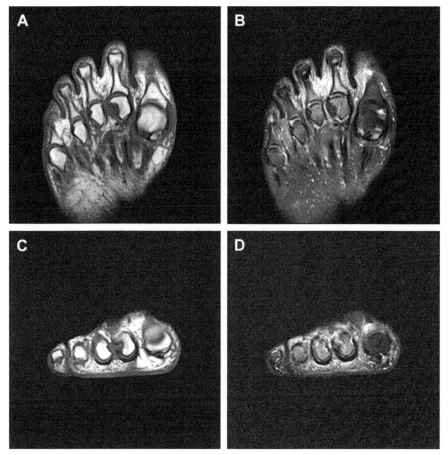

Fig. 1. MRI T1-weighted and T2-weighted axial (*A, B*) and coronal (*C, D*) views of a BML of the second metatarsal head.

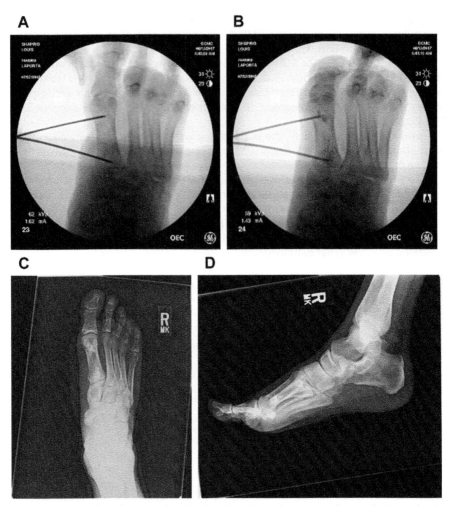

Fig. 2. Intraoperative photographs showing insertion of trocar and cannula in to the 1st metatarsal head and base (*A*), injection of the flowable CaP materials (*B*), and postoperative dorsoplantar and lateral radiographs (*C, D*).

REFERENCES

1. Curtiss PH Jr, Kincaid WE. Transitory demineralization of the hip in pregnancy. A report of three cases. J Bone Joint Surg Am 1959;41:1327–33.
2. Korompilias AV, Karantanas AH, Lykissas MG, et al. Bone marrow edema syndrome. Skeletal Radiol 2008;38(5):425–36.
3. Hofmann S, Kramer J, Vakil-Adli A, et al. Painful bone marrow edema of the knee: differential diagnosis and therapeutic concepts. Orthop Clin North Am 2004;35: 321–33.
4. Steinbach L, Suh K. Bone marrow edema pattern around the knee on magnetic resonance imaging excluding acute traumatic lesions. Semin Musculoskelet Radiol 2011;15(03):208–20.
5. Roemer FW, Frobell R, Hunter DJ, et al. MRI-detected subchondral bone marrow signal alterations of the knee joint: terminology, imaging appearance,

relevance and radiological diVerential diagnosis. Osteoarthr Cartil 2009;17(9): 1115–31.

6. Eriksen EF, Ringe JD. Bone marrow lesions: a universal bone response to injury? Rheumatol Int 2011;32(3):575–84.
7. Felson DT, Chaisson CE, Hill CL, et al. The association of bone marrow lesions with pain in knee osteoarthritis. Ann Intern Med 2001;134(7):541–9.
8. Valderrabano V, Horisberger M, Russell I, et al. Etiology of ankle arthritis. Clin Orthop Relat Res 2009;467(7):1800–6.
9. Ng A, Bernhard A, Bernhard K. Advances in ankle cartilage repair. Clin Podiatr Med Surg 2017;34(4):471–87.
10. Dijk CN, Reilingh ML, Zengerink M, et al. Osteochondral defects in the ankle: why painful? Knee Surg Sports Traumatol Arthrosc 2010;18(5):570–80.
11. Shepherd DE, Seedhom BB. Thickness of human articular cartilage in joints of the lower limb. Ann Rheum Dis 1999;58:27–34.
12. Qiu Y, Shahgaldi B, Revell W, et al. Observations of subchondral plate advancement during osteochondral repair: a histomorphometric and mechanical study in the rabbit femoral condyle. Osteoarthritis Cartilage 2003;11(11):810–20.
13. Sharkey P, Cohen S. Subchondroplasty for treating bone marrow lesions. J Knee Surg 2015;29(07):555–63.
14. Bonadio MB, Giglio PN, Helito CP, et al. Subchondroplasty for treating bone marrow lesions in the knee – initial experience. Rev Bras Ortop 2017;52(3): 325–30 (English Edition).
15. Miller JR, Dunn KW. Subchondroplasty of the ankle: a novel technique. The Foot and Ankle Online Journal 2015;8(1):1–7.

Resorbable Polymer Pin Inserted with Ultrasound Activated BoneWelding Technique Compared with a Screw for Osteotomy Fixation in the Reverse L Bunion Correction

Thomas M. Rocchio, DPM[a,b,*]

KEYWORDS

- Sonic pin • BoneWelding • Distal L bunionectomy • Bioresorbable • Polylactide pin
- Ultrasound activated • Hallux valgus • Osteoporosis

KEY POINTS

- Screw fixation of an osteotomy in the first metatarsal for bunion correction represents a compromise that includes anatomic restrictions, poor fixation in osteoporotic bone, and possible need for hardware removal surgery.
- A reversed L osteotomy for bunion repair combines the correction benefits of more proximal osteotomies with the stability of the distal chevron osteotomy.
- Bunion osteotomy fixation with an absorbable poly-DL lactic acid pin inserted with an ultrasound-activated BoneWelding technique eliminates future hardware retrieval surgery, minimizes undesirable inflammatory response, and is stable in osteoporotic bone.

INTRODUCTION

Surgical correction of a bunion deformity presents many considerations. Variations in osteotomy shape as well as the anatomic location that the osteotomy is performed creates not only differing levels of stability, but also a varying range of deformity correction that can be safely achieved. Additional considerations include the patient's ability to comply with the postoperative protocol. A patient with a larger bunion deformity who is independent and lives alone may not be able to follow a postoperative

Financial Disclosure: The author is a consultant for Stryker Orthopedics, Mahwah, NJ.
a PA Foot and Ankle Associates, 2895 Hamilton Boulevard, Suite 101, Allentown, PA 18104, USA; b Easton Hospital Wound Healing Center, 21 Community Drive, Easton, PA 18045, USA
* Corresponding author. 2895 Hamilton Boulevard, Suite 101, Allentown, PA 18104.
E-mail addresses: trocc8@gmail.com; trocchio@pafootdoctors.com

Clin Podiatr Med Surg 35 (2018) 373–385
https://doi.org/10.1016/j.cpm.2018.05.001
0891-8422/18/© 2018 Elsevier Inc. All rights reserved.

podiatric.theclinics.com

course that requires nonweightbearing. Osteotomies that are able to correct larger deformities may be less stable and would require a varying length of time nonweightbearing. The scarf is known for its correction ability, but is more technically demanding and more invasive than distal osteotomies.[1] The Chevron osteotomy is well-known and popular for its intrinsic stability and relative ease of performing. Over the past several decades, there has been interest in the corrective ability and the increased stability of the distal L bunionectomy.[2–8]

Studying the stiffness as well as the cortical bone strains and strength and failure mode of the scarf, chevron, and the reverse-L osteotomy with one author identifying that, "the critical weakening proximal apex of the scarf is avoided in the reverse-L, leading to results comparable to the chevron." The authors concluded that the reversed L osteotomy offers benefit of increased correction as seen in the scarf osteotomy and increased stability that is seen in the chevron.[4]

Another study compared the stability of the scarf, modified chevron, and reversed L osteotomies. The study showed that the total contact area of the chevron was 116 mm^2, the distal L was 163 mm^2, and the scarf was 270 mm^2, concluding that the reversed L osteotomy combines the advantage of both the chevron and scarf osteotomy.[5] Addressing the clinical presentation of the elderly patient with a large intermetatarsal angle that would normally be corrected with a proximal procedure, another study combined the distal L osteotomy with adductor tendon transfer that allowed a more tolerable postoperative protocol in this compromised population.[7]

Helmy and colleagues[6] studied the reversed L osteotomy for the correction of moderate and severe hallux valgus deformities with excellent clinical results noted in their 31-patient study. Loretz and colleagues[8] reviewed 69 distal L or Reverdin-Laird procedures with a high level of patient satisfaction at 94.2%.

The osteotomy performed by this author on the patients in this study represented most closely the Reverdin-Laird procedure (**Fig. 1**). A variation from the Laird modification was that a majority of the osteotomies performed did not incorporate a derotational wedge resection component. An additional variation from the Revirdin-Laird osteotomy that was consistent with all osteotomies performed was a significantly shorter dorsal osteotomy, necessitating a plantar cut that was not parallel to the weightbearing surface but still exited proximal to the sesamoid articulation.[9]

Once a decision of the best corrective osteotomy has been made, there is the need for selection of appropriate fixation. Although screws can be used to fixate most bunion osteotomy procedures, plates, pins (buried or percutaneous), cerclage wire,

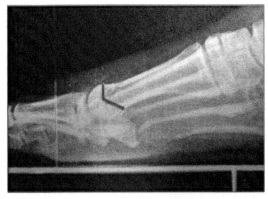

Fig. 1. Modified distal L osteotomy. Note the short dorsal osteotomy and longer plantar osteotomy angled to exit proximal to the sesamoid articulation.

absorbable products, and external fixation are all options. Although not unique in his thinking, the original description of the very popular chevron osteotomy described was without fixation.[10] With each different fixation option benefit there can be limitations and potential complications.

With respect to every different bunion correcting osteotomy, a fixation discussion could be extensive. The fixation discussion focuses on those options for the reverse L osteotomy. The placement of this osteotomy necessitates a dorsal proximal to plantar distal orientation that does not allow for bicortical screw purchase without invading the sesamoid articulation. Screw fixation with a headed cancellous screw is difficult to countersink without anatomic compromise and the head may become painful or palpable to the patient. Headless screws can be used but, in addition to the concern of plantar cortical breakthrough risk, these devices are not as stable as they are with a bicortical application. It is also this author's experience that cases of advanced osteopenia and cystic presentation also significantly reduce the effectiveness of the screw compression and stability of fixation.

Percutaneous K-wire placement for the stabilization of many distal first metatarsal osteotomies including the distal L bunion osteotomies offers a noncompressive alternative to screw placement. Although this author has used this technique, it is not a favorable option because there is varying stability and the addition of pin track irritation and infection as a possible complication.[8]

Absorbable pins and absorbable screws have been used for inherently stable bunion osteotomy fixation for many years with acceptable results.[11–18] Complications that are unique to absorbable material use include foreign body reaction, detritic synovitis, granuloma formation, sterile sinus tract, sterile abscess, bone resorption, and progressing osteoarthritis. A study focused on distal metatarsal osteotomies fixated with 2 different bioabsorbable implants. Of the 34 osteotomies fixated with a polydioxanon pin, 1 patient had a dorsal subluxed malunion compared with 11 osteotomies fixated with polyglycolide pins with findings in 6 of bone resorption and osteolytic event and 2 osteotomies with dorsal subluxed malunion.[19] Although this study found no foreign body reaction in their patient population, other articles report cases of foreign body reaction from poly-p-dioxanon pin use.[20,21]

Just over the past decade, a polylactide polymer has been inserted with an ultrasonic BoneWelding technique. The ultrasonic energy applied to the resorbable Sonic Pin (Stryker, Mahwah, NJ) resulted in a liquefaction that allowed the polymer to flow into the porous structures of the cancellous bone and then harden in several seconds to form a 3-dimensional fixation (**Fig. 2**).

The polymer used in the BoneWelding technique is made of poly-L-lactic acid that has been safely used for several decades.[22,23] This polymer has properties that distinguish it from other absorbable implants. Possessing a significantly slower resorption profile that is measured in years, the use of a poly-L-lactic acid implant produced a lesser inflammatory response and eliminated cystic changes or osteolysis. Slower resorption also allowed for a maintained mechanical strength of the implant of 30 weeks.[24–26] It has been researched that the thermal stress that ultrasonic BoneWelding techniques induce did not lead to any cellular reaction in the bone with finding of new bone formation observed without inflammatory reaction.[26,27]

The Sonic Pin (Stryker), inserted through a predrilled hole with BoneWelding technology, was developed to address cancellous bone fixation needs. In both stable and osteoporotic human cadaver bone, the polymeric implant inserted with the BoneWelding technique showed superior anchoring when compared with metal screws.[28,29] This technique and product have been used safely in foot and ankle surgical fixation for more than 10 years.[30–33]

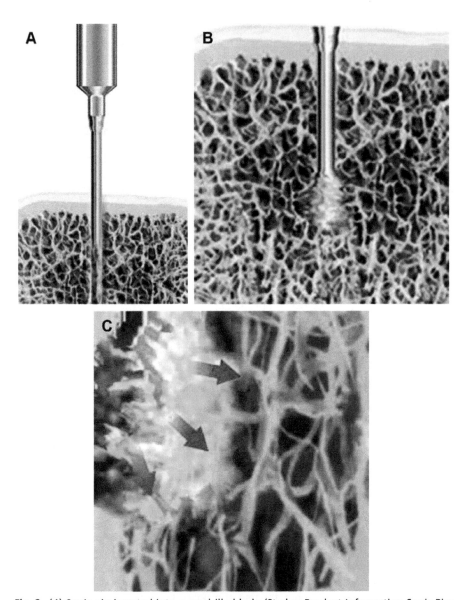

Fig. 2. (*A*) Sonic pin inserted into a predrilled hole (Stryker Product Information Sonic Pin: Literature number: B1000086-US Rev 0/11). (*B*) Sonic Pin liquefied at the tip with the introduction of ultrasonic energy causing interdigitation into the porous structure of cancellous bone. (*C*) Cooling of polymer after interdigitation provides a solid 3-dimensional structure. (*Courtesy of* Stryker, Mahwah, NJ; with permission.)

A similar study used MRI to evaluate this polymer's resorption behavior after a chevron bunionectomy with no findings of foreign body reaction occurring after 12 months and no visible signs of resorption of the implant.[31] A similar study with postoperative MRI that extended further demonstrated all 25 osteotomies studied healed without adverse reaction, all having implants still visible at the 36-month MRI, and 14 of the 25 having complete resorption of the implant at 48 months.[34]

Materials and Methods

A consecutive series of patients with painful moderate to severe bunion deformity treated with a modified distal L osteotomy for correction were reviewed. Patient records were evaluated for demographic information, severity of deformity, type of osteotomy fixation used, complications, need for additional surgical procedure, and patient satisfaction. Two distinct groups were identified for comparison. The first group had a Distal L osteotomy fixated with a 4.0 small frag screw (Synthes, West Chester, PA). The second group had the same osteotomy fixation with the bioresorbable (poly L-lactide-co-D, L-lactide 70:30) Sonic Pin (Stryker) inserted using an ultrasonic BoneWelding technique.

Patient Selection and Preoperative Protocol

All patients selected for this procedure presented with a history of painful bunion deformity that was nonresponsive to conservative treatments. This conservative treatment included attempts at orthotic management, proper fitting shoes, protective shields and spacers, nonsteroidal anti-inflammatory drugs, steroid injection, and physical therapy.

All patients received a full biomechanical examination and radiographic examination that included radiographic deformity assessment. The intermetatarsal angle and hallux valgus angle were included in the measurements to determine osteotomy variation, such as the addition of a trapezoidal wedge to derotate the articular cartilage. A final decision on the use of this variation was made with examination of the exposed joint during surgery.

Surgical Technique

All of the procedures in this study were performed by the same surgeon. The standard procedure for every patient was performed using a dorsal medial incision over the first metatarsal head that was medial to the extensor halluces longus and carried across the metatarsal phalangeal joint. A T-shaped capsulotomy was created and the joint was exposed. Lateral release was performed if necessary and the medial prominence was resected. A 0.045 K-wire was inserted as a guide from medial to lateral across the distal metatarsal head approximately 4 mm proximal from the end of the dorsal articular cartilage and approximately 4 to 5 mm plantar from the dorsal surface of the metatarsal. An L-shaped osteotomy was created from medial to lateral with the dorsal cut perpendicular to the weightbearing surface and the longer plantar cut angled to exit the first metatarsal proximal to the articulation with the sesamoids (see **Fig. 1**). If deemed necessary, a dorsal derotational osteotomy was created just proximal to the original dorsal osteotomy with base medial and apex lateral to remove a dorsal wedge to facilitate joint space rotation. The capital fragment was shifted lateral and temporarily fixated with a 0.045 K-wire from dorsal proximal to plantar distal, catching the most medial portion of the capital fragment (**Fig. 3**).

Technique Variation for Group I

Once the desired correction was obtained and the temporary fixation was stable, a 2.5-mm drill was used to create a guide hole across the osteotomy from dorsal proximal to plantar distal. Care was then taken to countersink this dorsal cortical bone in an attempt to reduce hardware irritation postoperatively. A depth gauge was then used for screw length determination and a 4.0 tap was inserted. Finally a single 4.0 mm cancellous screw (Synthes) was inserted (**Fig. 4**).

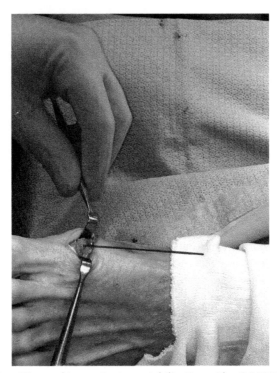

Fig. 3. Corrected position and transosteotomy stabilization with a 0.045 K-wire placed from proximal dorsal to distal medial into the medial metatarsal head.

Technique Variation for Group II

Once the desired correction was obtained and the temporary fixation was stable, a 0.8 mm × 100 mm K-wire was placed across the osteotomy from dorsal proximal to plantar distal into the distal fragment using visual or intraoperative imaging with care taken not to advance the K-wire through the distal cortical bone (**Fig. 5**). A dedicated depth gauge was used to measure for appropriate pin length and associated cannulated drill was then used to create the guide hole for the polymer pin (**Fig. 6**). It is important to note that, when using this system, the dedicated drill for the desired pin length will create a countersink for the polymer head and that the guide hole is 6 to 8 mm shorter than the length of the pin to allow for adequate liquification and advancement of the polymer pin during ultrasonic insertion.

The Sonic Pin (Stryker) was mounted onto the sonotrode hand piece and inserted into the guide hole (**Fig. 7**). Placing a mild axial force on the pin loaded on the hand piece, a foot pedal was pressed to initiate the ultrasonic energy producing liquification of the tip of the pin until it was fully seated (**Fig. 8**). Release of the foot pedal halted the ultrasonic energy and in 5 seconds an audible signal indicated the surgeon was clear to remove the hand piece from the fully seated pin.

Removal of the temporary 0.045 K-wire, resection of remaining dorsal medial shelf of bone, appropriate capsular work, and primary soft tissue closure was then performed on both groups of patients. The postoperative protocol for all patients included a surgical splinted dressing with full weight bearing allowed in a pneumatic walking boot for 4 weeks. Radiographs were performed immediately postoperatively and at regular follow-up visits at 2 weeks, 6 weeks, 3 months, and 6 months.

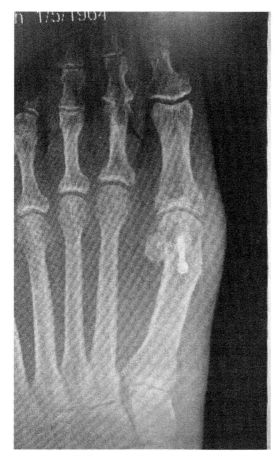

Fig. 4. Postoperative radiograph demonstrating osteotomy fixation with a 4.0 cancellous screw.

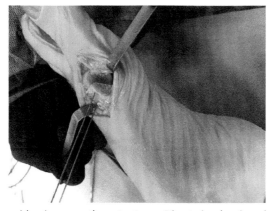

Fig. 5. An 0.8-mm guide pin across the osteotomy. Direct visual or imaging can be used for optimal placement with care not to drill through the plantar cortical bone.

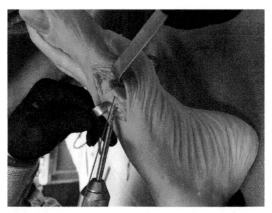

Fig. 6. After measuring for pin length the designated cannulated drill over the 0.8-mm guide pin.

Results

In this retrospective consecutive series, 356 distal L osteotomy bunion correction surgeries were performed on 272 patients between October 2003 and February 2017. This series of patients was further divided into 2 groups, with the first group receiving osteotomy fixation with a single 4.0 cancellous screw and the second group receiving osteotomy fixation with a resorbable polymer pin (poly-L-lactide-co-D, L-lactide 70:30) inserted with ultrasonic BoneWelding technology.

Group patients 1 (4.0 screw fixation) underwent 183 procedures with a procedural population of 142 female and 41 male with average age of 44.2 years (range, 14–72 years) at the time of surgery. Of the 183 patient procedures, 44 included derotational wedge resection. There were no nonunions in this group. Two of the patients had a dorsal shift of the capital fragment with malunion that did not necessitate revisional procedure. There were 11 cases of superficial skin dehiscence treated successfully in the clinic with 15 patients receiving oral antibiotic from superficial cellulitis with no effect on final result. Three patients had intraoperative inadequate fixation with lack

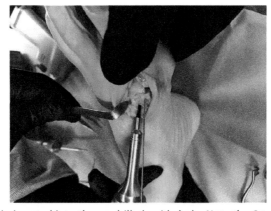

Fig. 7. Polymer pin inserted into the predrilled guide hole. Note the 6 to 8 mm exposed to allow for polymer flow into the porous structures of the cancellous bone on insertion.

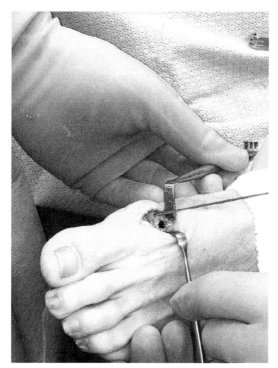

Fig. 8. Fully seated polymer pin after insertion with the ultrasonic BoneWelding technique. Note the flush low profile after insertion aided by the countersink component of the guide hole drill.

of screw purchase that necessitated additional percutaneous temporary pin fixation. There were 72 patients who required additional surgical hardware removal owing to pain. Overall patient satisfaction was 91.5% based on elimination of pain and correction of deformity.

Group 2 patients (polymer pin fixation with ultrasonic BoneWelding technology) underwent 173 procedures with a procedural population of 138 females and 35 males with an average age of 43.6 years (range, 16–73 years) at the time of surgery. Of these patients, 69 underwent an additional derotational wedge resection. In this group, there were no nonunions and no dorsal shifting with no malunions. There were 6 dehiscence events treated successfully in the clinic with 15 patients receiving a prescription for an oral antibiotic for superficial cellulitis with no effect on final postoperative result. None of these patients had lack of fixation purchase intraoperatively and none of these patients required additional internal fixation of any kind. None of these patients required an additional surgical procedure. Overall patient satisfaction was 91.3% based on elimination of pain and correction of deformity (**Fig. 9**).

Discussion

Osteotomy selection for the correction of a bunion deformity depends on more than just the size of the deformity. Procedures to correct a larger bunion deformity, such as the scarf procedure, historically require more dissection, are more technically difficult to perform, and result in a less stable construct that could require an longer period of nonweightbearing.[1] Distal head procedures, such as the chevron osteotomy, are

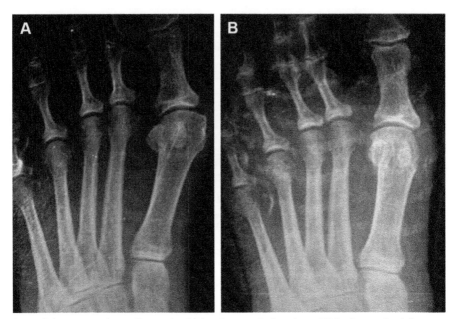

Fig. 9. (*A*) Preoperative radiograph of a bunion surgical patient. (*B*) Radiograph of the same patient after operative correction with Distal L osteotomy fixated by insertion of an ultrasonic liquified polymer pin.

inherently stable but may not allow adequate correction of a larger deformity.[10] The reversed (or distal) L osteotomy has been shown to represent a stable construct in the distal metatarsal that can also provide increased correction.[2–8]

Studies comparing the chevron, scarf, and the reverse L osteotomy show significantly increased total bone contact area of the reversed L when compared with the chevron procedure, concluding that reverse L osteotomy combined the advantage of both the chevron and the scarf osteotomies.[5] An additional study focused on the use of the reverse L osteotomy in a compromised elderly population with satisfactory postoperative results and a noted benefit from a more tolerable postoperative protocol.[7]

The fixation of an osteotomy in the first metatarsal for bunion correction with screws represents a compromise. The need to return to the operating room for removal exposes patients to added anesthesia risk and expense, as well as the addition of potential common surgical complications. In this study, the osteotomies fixated with a screw required an additional screw removal surgery in 39.3% of cases. Screw fixation is also limited by anatomic restrictions. Screw fixation in the reversed L osteotomy requires cancellous screw that performs less than satisfactorily in osteoporotic bone or in the presence of cysts in the head of the metatarsal. Three patients reviewed in this article who underwent screw fixation required additional percutaneous pin fixation owing to inadequate screw fixation and 2 other screw-fixated osteotomies suffered dorsal shift and malunion.

Although absorbable pin and screw fixation of osteotomies has been favorably reported for many years,[11–18] this form of fixation has been plagued with product-specific complications that include foreign body reaction, detritic synovitis, granuloma, sterile sinus tract, sterile abscess, bone resorption, and osteoarthritis.[19–21]

Distinguishing itself from other resorbable implants, the Sonic Pin (Stryker) is made of poly L-lactide-co-D, L-lactide in a 70:30 ratio that allows this polymer pin to maintained mechanical strength for 30 weeks with a significantly slower resorption rate, resulting in a lesser inflammatory response and the elimination of cystic changes or osteolysis.[24–26] Inserted with ultrasonic BoneWelding techniques provides a stable 3-dimensional fixation with a liquification of the tip of the pin into the porous structures of cancellous bone and near immediate solidification without measurable damage to the surrounding bone or tissue and without inflammatory reaction.[26,27]

When compared with the series of osteotomies fixated with a screw, there were no Sonic Pin (Stryker) fixated osteotomies that required additional fixation owing to operative instability and there were no cases of osteotomy dorsal shifting or subsequent malunion. Of greatest note, none of the patients in this group required a return to the operating arena because no retrieval of the resorbable pin was ever necessary.

The process of ultrasonic polymer pin insertion is ideal for fixation in compromised osteoporotic and cystic bone when compared with screws. Liquification of the polymer into this porous bone creates stability in an already unstable anatomy with an interdigitated 3-dimensional solidified construct.

SUMMARY

Bunion correction by means of a reversed L osteotomy fixated with the ultrasonic BoneWelding technique with the Sonic Pin (Stryker) offers surgical patients a more tolerable postoperative course and elimination of the risk of undergoing an additional hardware retrieval surgery. This procedure also offers the surgeon a solution for the correction of symptomatic bunion deformity in the compromised osteoporotic patient by using a unique welding technique combined with the stability of reverse L osteotomy, allowing a less aggressive postoperative recovery period.

REFERENCES

1. Zygmunt KH, Gudas CJ, Laros GS. Z-bunionectomy with internal screw fixation. J Am Podiatr Med Assoc 1989;79(7):322–9.
2. Chudy DE, DiMaggio JA. Bicorrectional horizontal v-osteotomy of the first metatarsal head. J Foot Surg 1983;22(3):226–9.
3. Zyzda MJ, Hineser W. Distal L osteotomy in treatment of hallux abducto valgus. J Foot Surg 1989;28(5):445–8.
4. Favre P, Farine M, Snedeker JG, et al. Biomechanical consequences of first metatarsal osteotomy in treating hallux valgus. Clin Biomech (Bristol, Avon) 2010; 25(7):721–7.
5. Vienne P, Favre P, Meyer D, et al. Comparative mechanical testing of different geometric designs of distal first metatarsal osteotomies. Foot Ankle Int 2007; 28(2):232–6.
6. Helmy N, Vienne P, Von Came A, et al. Treatment of hallux valgus deformity: preliminary results with a modified distal metatarsal osteotomy. Acta Orthop Belg 2009;75(5):661–70.
7. Vega MR, Jackson-Smith JL. A variable first metatarsal distal L osteotomy with adductor tendon transfer. J Foot Ankle Surg 1995;34(4):384–8.
8. Loretz L, DeValentine S, Yamaguchi K. The first metatarsal bicorrectional head osteotomy (disml "L"/Reverdin-Laird procedure) for correction of hallux abducto valgus: a retrospective study. J Foot Ankle Surg 1993;32:554–68.
9. Laird PO, Silvers SH, Somdahl J. Two Reverdin-Laird osteotomy modifications or correction of hallux abducto valgus. J Am Podiatr Med Assoc 1988;78:403–5.

10. Austin DW, Leventen EO. A new osteotomy for the hallux valgus: a horizontally directed "V" displacement osteotomy of the metatarsal head for hallux valgus and primus varus. Clin Orthop 1981;157:25–30.
11. Brunetti VA, Trepal MJ, Jules KT. Fixation of the Austin osteotomy with bioresorbable pins. J Foot Surg 1991;30(1):56–65.
12. Gerber J. Effectiveness of absorbable fixation devices in Austin bunionectomies. J Am Podiatr Med Assoc 1992;82(4):189–95.
13. Hetherington VJ, Shields SL, Wilhelm KR, et al. Absorbable fixation of the first ray osteotomies. J Foot Ankle Surg 1994;33(3):290–4.
14. Friends GJ, Grace KS, Stone HA. Cortical screws versus absorbable pins for fixation of the short Z-bunionectomy. J Foot Ankle Surg 1994;33(4):411–8.
15. Gill LH, Martin DF, Coumas JM, et al. Fixation with bioabsorbable pins in chevron bunionectomy. J Bone Joint Surg Am 1997;79:1510–8.
16. Caminear DS, Pavlovich R Jr, Pietrzak WS. Fixation of the chevron osteotomy with an absorbable copolymer pin for treatment of hallux valgus deformity. J Foot Ankle Surg 2005;44(3):203–10.
17. Alcelik I, Alnaib M, Pollock R, et al. Bioabsorbable fixation for Mitchell's bunionectomy osteotomy. J Foot Ankle Surg 2009;48(1):9–14.
18. Morandi A, Ungaro E, Fraccia A, et al. Chevron osteotomy of the first metatarsal stabilized with an absorbable pin: our 5-year experience. Foot Ankle Int 2013; 34(3):380–5.
19. Lavery LA, Peterson JD, Pollack R, et al. Risk of complications of first metatarsal head osteotomies with biodegradable pin fixation: biofix versus orthosorb. J Foot Ankle Surg 1994;33(4):334–40.
20. Kalla TP, Janzen DL. Orthosorb: a case of foreign-body reaction. J Foot Ankle Surg 1995;34(4):366–70.
21. Frederick J, Hulst TJ, Sundareson AS. Foreign-body reaction to absorbable fixation devices. J Am Podiatr Med Assoc 1996;86(8):396–8.
22. Leenslag JW, Pennings AJ, Bos RR, et al. Resorbable materials of poly(L-Lactide). VI. plates and screws for internal fixation fracture fixation. Biomaterials 1987;8(1):70–3.
23. Barca F, Busa R. Austin/chevron osteotomy fixed with bioabsorbable poly-L-lactic acid single screw. J Foot Ankle Surg 1997;36(1):15–20.
24. Claes LE, Ignatius AA, Rehm KE, et al. New bioresorbable pin for the reduction of small bony fragments: designs, mechanical properties and in vitro degradation. Biomaterials 1996;17(16):1621–6.
25. Claes L, Ignatius A. Development of new, biodegradable implants. Chirurg 2002; 73(10):990–6.
26. Mai R, Lauer G, Pilling E, et al. Bone welding – a histologic evaluation in the jaw. Ann Anat 2007;189(4):350–5.
27. Langhoff JD, Kuemmerle JM, Mayer J, et al. An ultrasound assisted anchoring technique (BoneWelding® Technology) for fixation of implants to bone – a histological pilot study in sheep. Open Orthop J 2009;3:40–7.
28. Feruson SJ, Weber U, von Rechenberg B, et al. Enhancing the mechanical integrity of the implant-bone interface with bone welding technology: determination of quasi-static interface strength and fatigue resistance. J Biomed Mater Res B Appl Biomater 2006;77(1):13–20.
29. Meyer DC, Mayer J, Weber U, et al. Ultrasonically implanted PLA suture anchors are stable in osteopenic bone. Clin Orthop Relat Res 2006;442:143–8.
30. Rocchio T. A Closer look at the corrective potential of ultrasonic bone-welding®. Podiatry Today 2017;30(1):1–2.

31. Olms K, Randt T, Reimers N, et al. Ultrasonic assisted anchoring of biodegradable implants for chevron osteotomies – clinical evaluation of a novel fixation method. Open Orthop J 2014;8:85–92.
32. Rocchio T, Kruger A, Grahm B. Lesser metatarsal decompression osteotomy fixation with an ultrasonic bioresorbable polymer pin utilizing bone welding® principles. Las Vegas (NV): ACFAS Poster; 2017.
33. Rocchio T, Grahm B, Kruger A. Fixation of the opening wedge calcaneal osteotomy with ultrasonic bioresorbable polymer pin utilizing bone welding® principle. Las Vegas (NV): ACFAS Poster; 2017.
34. Olms K, Arrington, JA, Reimers N, et al. Resorption characteristics of a PLDLLA implant inserted with ultrasonic energy-results from four year follow-up. Poster.

Minimally Invasive Bunion Correction

Noman A. Siddiqui, DPM, MHA[a],*, Guido A. LaPorta, DPM, MS[b,c]

KEYWORDS

- Minimally invasive • Percutaneous • Triplanar • Bunion correction • Hallux valgus
- Bunion deformity

KEY POINTS

- Hallux valgus has been treated surgically with an open technique for many years, which involves open soft-tissue balancing and osteotomy with internal fixation to realign the malaligned toe.
- Percutaneous/minimally invasive methods are growing in popularity for many orthopedic procedures, including hallux valgus.
- Minimally invasive surgery allows for faster recovery, decreased operating time, cosmetic scarring, and equivalent healing compared with open procedures reported in the literature.
- This method can be applied to a variety of hallux valgus deformities (mild, moderate, severe) to achieve an excellent outcome.

INTRODUCTION

Hallux valgus is a common forefoot condition that can be described as mild, moderate, or severe. It is characterized by lateral deviation and pronation of the hallux and medial deviation of the first metatarsal. This progressive condition can lead to pain with ambulation, difficulty with shoe gear, soft-tissue irritation (digital neuritis/bursitis), transfer plantar lesser metatarsal lesions, and digital deformities. Constrictive shoe gear and a genetic predisposition have been implicated as extrinsic and intrinsic factors in the development of this condition.[1–6] If conservative measures to manage this painful condition fail, surgical intervention is used to realign the great toe joint.

Traditional approaches to mild to moderate hallux valgus correction have been described as open approaches that consist of single or multiple incisions that involve capsular dissection, resection of the medial eminence, release of lateral ligamentous

Disclosure Statement: The authors have nothing to disclose.
[a] International Center for Limb Lengthening, Rubin Institute for Advanced Orthopedics, Sinai Hospital of Baltimore, 2401 West Belvedere Avenue, Baltimore, MD 21215, USA; [b] Geisinger CMC, 1800 Mulberry St, Scranton, PA 18510, USA; [c] Our Lady of Lourdes Memorial Hospital, 169 Riverside Dr, Binghamton, NY 13905, USA
* Corresponding author.
E-mail address: nsiddiqu@lifebridgehealth.org

Clin Podiatr Med Surg 35 (2018) 387–402
https://doi.org/10.1016/j.cpm.2018.05.002
0891-8422/18/© 2018 Elsevier Inc. All rights reserved.

podiatric.theclinics.com

and tendinous structures, capsule tendon balancing, and placement of internal fixation.[6,7] Severe deformities involve correction with more proximal metatarsal osteotomies and/or metatarsal-cuneiform fusion.[8] An abundance of articles exist on these open methods of correction that report good to excellent radiographic outcomes with high patient satisfaction rates.[9,10]

In comparison, there seems to be a relative paucity of literature that has looked at outcomes with a minimal or percutaneous approach to correct hallux valgus.

Bösch and colleagues[11] were one of the first to describe and publish a minimally invasive approach to hallux valgus correction. This method used a small incision (<1 cm) over the metatarsal head and neck. Dissection was extended to the bone, and a Lindemann burr was used to complete the subcapital osteotomy. A grooved device was used to translate the metatarsal head into a corrected position, and a 2-mm Steinmann pin was placed into the medullary canal.[11] No additional soft-tissue procedures were performed. Bösch and colleagues[12] later reported results after following patients for 7 to 10 years who underwent the Bösch method of correction. In this study,[12] they reported the results of 4 different surgeons performing the procedure in 114 feet. Bösch and colleagues[12] reported excellent radiographic outcomes and a patient satisfaction rate of 81%. Patients also reported a 95% satisfaction rate at the long-term follow-up.

In North America, Isham[13] reported his minimally invasive modification to the Reverdin open method of bunion correction. The Reverdin-Isham modification method placed multiple small incisions at the level of the first metatarsophalangeal joint (MPJ). A small Shannon No. 44 burr was first introduced into the capsule to remove and reduce the medial eminence. A closing wedge osteotomy of the first metatarsal was performed through this same incision. A secondary incision was then made over the dorsal lateral aspect of the first MPJ, and a modified lateral release was performed. Finally, a third incision was made as needed at the level of the first proximal phalanx to complete an Akin osteotomy. No fixation was used, and the reduction was maintained with aggressive splinting and bandages.

Giannini and colleagues,[14] in 2003, described an alternative approach to percutaneous distal metatarsal osteotomy for hallux valgus. The approach varied in its method from Bösch and colleagues[11] by the manner of performing the osteotomy and fixating the capital fragment. Giannini and colleagues[14] performed a subcapital osteotomy with a saw (vs burr) and advanced the Steinmann pin retrograde through the incision toward the end of the digit before manipulating the pin into the medullary canal and advancing it into the metatarsal for stability.

Magnan and colleagues[15] similarly performed a distal first metatarsal osteotomy via a minimal incisional approach. They used the surgical method described by Bösch and colleagues[11,12] and reported radiographic and satisfaction outcomes for 118 feet. They observed improvement in all radiographic parameters, and 91% of patients were satisfied with the clinical results at the short-term follow-up.

Brogan and colleagues,[16] more recently, described a third-generation percutaneous correction. Brogan and colleagues[16] categorized the various approaches to minimally invasive bunion correction as first, second, and third generation. The first-generation technique uses medullary pin fixation as described by Bösch and colleagues.[11] Second-generation procedures used a chevron and akin osteotomy with internal fixation. The third-generation bunionectomy, by Brogan and colleagues,[16] used a hybrid of methods combining a medullary pin with internal fixation. They analyzed 45 feet and performed a minimally invasive chevron osteotomy at the metatarsal neck through a 5-mm incision. The chevron osteotomy was completed with a Shannon burr; the capital fragment was translated, as described by Bösch and colleagues,[11] and secured with 1.8-mm titanium medullary pin. The investigators then placed a headless screw 2 cm proximal to the initial skin incision. They reported clinically significant improvement in radiographic and patient satisfaction parameters.

However, there seems to be a steep learning curve with these methods.[15,17,18] Surgeons performing this method have advocated for additional cadaveric training and adherence to the surgical technique to prevent complications.[15,17,18] The authors of this article have been using the minimally invasive bunion correction method for many years[19] and have performed more than 300 procedures. The authors have added minor modifications to the technique described by Giannini and colleagues[14] and Magnan and colleagues,[15] yet have ensured application of the main principles of performing correction via a minimally invasive method for mild, moderate, and severe bunion deformities. The goal of this article is to provide surgeons with

- Indications/contraindications
- A systematic, detailed method to perform the correction
- Principles of correction
- Case examples

INDICATIONS AND CONTRAINDICATIONS

Indications to perform the osteotomy are patients

- With mild, moderate, and severe hallux valgus radiographically[13,20]
- With or without hypermobility
- With little or no arthritis

Contraindications are limited to

- Those with a history of bony or soft-tissue infections of the first MPJ
- Significant arthritis of the first MPJ
- Vascular compromise
- Recent distal open bunionectomy (<1 year)

SURGICAL TECHNIQUE

Patients are placed on the table in a supine position with a bump in a foot-forward position. It is important to allow the knee to bend to a 45° position to provide ease in obtaining anteroposterior (AP) view radiographs (**Fig. 1**A). The foot is prepped and draped in a standard aseptic manner, and regional and/or general anesthesia is

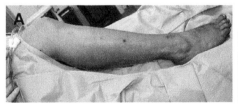
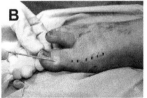

Fig. 1. (*A*) Clinical position before correction. Note that the knee is bent at 45°. (*B*) Pin started at the proximal corner of the nail. A traditional dorsal medial incision has been drawn for comparison with the small medial incision (<1 cm). (*C*) Steinmann pin (2-mm diameter) is inserted distally and advanced to the proximal aspect of the first MPJ. It is important to maintain good bony apposition as the pin is advanced to the MPJ. (*Courtesy of* Rubin Institute for Advanced Orthopedics, Sinai Hospital of Baltimore, Baltimore, MD. Copyright 2018.)

administered. When possible, and not contraindicated by the anesthesia service, the surgeons' preference is to use a regional ankle block with sedation. Two surgical perspectives are provided next.

PERSPECTIVE 1 (METHOD USED BY N.A.S.)
Step 1

A 2-mm Steinmann pin is inserted 2 to 3 mm from the medial proximal corner of the toenail of the first toe to the first MPJ (**Fig. 1**B, C).

Step 2

A 1-cm or smaller incision is made on the medial aspect of the first metatarsal, and blunt dissection is performed. The path of the osteotomy is directed by placing multiple drill holes with a bayonet tip 1.8-mm Ilizarov wire in a dorsal to plantar manner (corticotomy technique) (**Fig. 2**). The surgeon is able to angulate the guidewire to create an oblique osteotomy in the frontal plane to lengthen, shorten, or maintain a neutral length (after translation of the distal fragment). The osteotomy is completed with a small osteotome or a sagittal saw (**Fig. 3**).

Step 3

After the osteotomy is completed, a small hemostat or grooved device (Bösch instrument) was used to translate the capital fragment laterally (**Fig. 4**A). Simultaneously, a 2.0-mm Steinmann pin is placed into the medullary canal of the first metatarsal. The amount of this translation is allowed to be as great as 90% of the metaphyseal diaphyseal metatarsal shaft width (**Fig. 4**B–D). The goal is to maintain bony contact between the cortices.

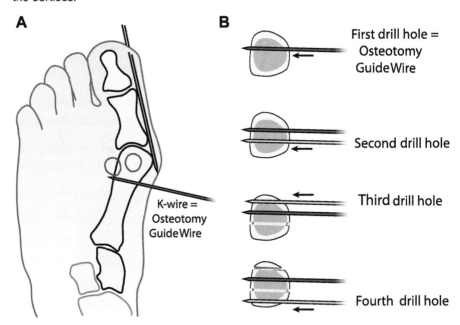

Fig. 2. (A) An initial guidewire is placed. This placement can be in the path of the osteotomy. (B) Multiple drill holes created above and below the guidewire along path of the osteotomy. K-wire, Kirschner wire. (*Courtesy of* Rubin Institute for Advanced Orthopedics, Sinai Hospital of Baltimore, Baltimore, MD. Copyright 2018.)

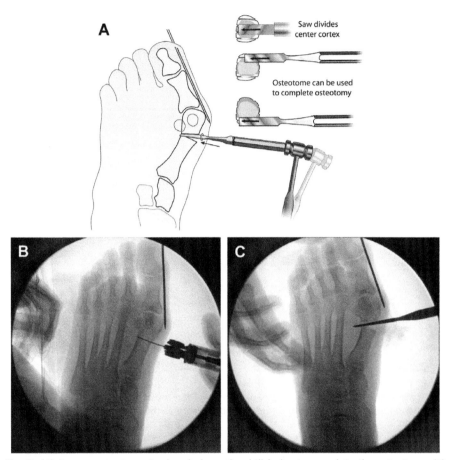

Fig. 3. (*A*) Saw or osteotome is placed along the drill holes to complete the osteotomy. (*B*) Intraoperative view shows a saw being used to complete the osteotomy. (*C*) Intraoperative view shows a small osteotome being used to complete the osteotomy. (*Courtesy of* Rubin Institute for Advanced Orthopedics, Sinai Hospital of Baltimore, Baltimore, MD. Copyright 2018.)

Step 4

The head of the first metatarsal is derotated (supinated) and translated (dorsal/plantar) in the frontal, transverse, and sagittal planes as needed to obtain reduction of the sesamoid apparatus and restore the articular surface congruency in all planes. Once correction is obtained, the Steinmann pin is advanced into the metatarsal-cuneiform joint for additional stability (see **Fig. 4**C, D).

Step 5

Excessive metatarsal bony protuberance should be rongeured through the same skin incision and the skin closed (**Fig. 4**E).

PERSPECTIVE 2 (METHOD USED BY G.L.)
Step 1

A 1-cm incision is made on the medial aspect of the first metatarsal, at the level of the metatarsal neck (metaphyseal-diaphyseal junction). Blunt dissection is carried down

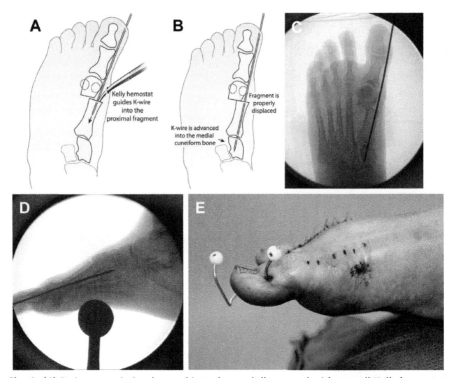

Fig. 4. (*A*) Steinmann pin is advanced into the medullary canal with a small Kelly hemostat. (*B*) Capital fragment is translated laterally. Any rotation is corrected before advancing the Steinmann pin into the metatarsal. (*C*) Pin is advanced into the medial cuneiform for stability. (*D*) Pin is centered in the metatarsal to maintain neutral dorsal and plantar translation. A dorsally placed pin will translate the head plantar and vice versa. (*E*) Cosmetic medial incision. K-wire, Kirschner wire. (*Courtesy of* Rubin Institute for Advanced Orthopedics, Sinai Hospital of Baltimore, Baltimore, MD. Copyright 2018.)

to the metatarsal neck. Dorsal periosteal elevation is performed with a small iris scissor or hemostat. The osteotomy is completed with a sagittal saw.

Step 2

After the osteotomy is completed, the Steinmann pin is placed through the incision and advanced antegrade toward the distal aspect of the toe and then retrograde through the medullary canal. The 2.0-mm Steinmann pin is manipulated to enter the medullary canal of the first metatarsal.

Step 3

The sesamoids are reduced, and the metatarsal head is stabilized with the medullary pin. The remainder of the method is similar to perspective 1.

Postoperative Protocol

Patients are encouraged to begin immediate weight bearing in a flat, rigid postoperative shoe. The bandage is removed 1 week after surgery, and normal showering is allowed. The postoperative shoe is maintained for 4 weeks, at which point the pin is removed in the clinic. Patients are transitioned to wearing a sturdy sneaker to start normal weight bearing. Patients are given range-of-motion (ROM) exercises that focus primarily on dorsiflexion and plantarflexion of the great toe joint (**Fig. 5**A). Radiographs are obtained during follow-up visits until consolidation is confirmed at the osteotomy site. Light exercise is resumed at 8 weeks with normal impact sports usually permitted after the 3-month follow-up visit. Patients can usually resume full activity at 10 to 12 weeks or when bony consolidation is noted (**Fig. 5**B, C).

PRINCIPLES OF CORRECTION

When performing an osteotomy with the minimal incision or percutaneous approach, the surgeon should follow these principles to ensure excellent healing:

- Ensure minimal soft-tissue disruption
- Preserve vascularity
- Obtain anatomic reduction and mechanical realignment
- Maintain relative stability of the osteotomy
- Encourage early mobilization of the MPJ

Ensure Minimal Soft-Tissue Disruption

Open bunionectomy procedures are used to address osseous and soft-tissue components that contribute to the development of the deformity. In general, most bunionectomy procedures will have a soft-tissue release of the medial and lateral capsule and ligamentous attachments. A medial capsulotomy/capsulorrhaphy along with aggressive release of the tibial sesamoid ligaments are considered imperative for correction. A secondary incision over the first interspace to perform a lateral release of the tendinous, capsular, and fibular sesamoid ligaments has been extensively described.[6,7] However, these steps are completely omitted when performing a minimally invasive approach. There is no capsular or ligamentous release performed

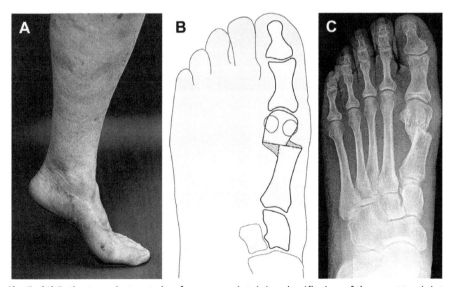

Fig. 5. (*A*) Patients are instructed to focus on maintaining dorsiflexion of the great toe joint. Note the small medial incision on the first metatarsal. (*B*) Bony union occurs along the path of the realigned metatarsal head. (*C*) At 1 year after correction, bony remodeling was noted as well as radiographic alignment of the first ray. (*Courtesy of* Rubin Institute for Advanced Orthopedics, Sinai Hospital of Baltimore, Baltimore, MD. Copyright 2018.)

on the medial or lateral soft-tissue attachments to the metatarsal head and base of the proximal phalanx. This lack of release reduces the incisional approach needed to obtain correction. The initial 5- to 10-mm skin incision is used to dissect full thickness in an extracapsular manner to the bone. The soft-tissue ligamentous and tendinous attachments remain around the MPJ, thus, allowing circumferential mobility to reduce the sesamoid apparatus into the appropriate anatomic location (**Fig. 6**).

Preserve Vascularity

Avascular necrosis of the metatarsal head is a rare complication during distal bunionectomy procedures. By limiting the soft-tissue dissection in minimally invasive bunionectomy, there are inherent vascular benefits to the metatarsal head. Maintaining the capsular attachments preserves the vascular supply to the metatarsal. Minimal periosteal dissection is performed before the osteotomy (as described in the surgical technique), which further promotes robust healing.

Obtain Anatomic Reduction and Mechanical Realignment

With the minimal invasive method of correction, obtaining anatomic reduction can be challenging because of the visual limitations and lack of surgical exposure. The surgeon must rely heavily on C-arm fluoroscopy to ensure that after the osteotomy is performed, the capital fragment maintains the appropriate reduction. Reduction of the sesamoid apparatus and MPJ in the transverse and frontal plane with appropriate dorsal/plantar translation will optimize healing and postrecovery function. The realignment of the mechanical axis will improve ROM and decrease deforming forces on the joint.[21,22]

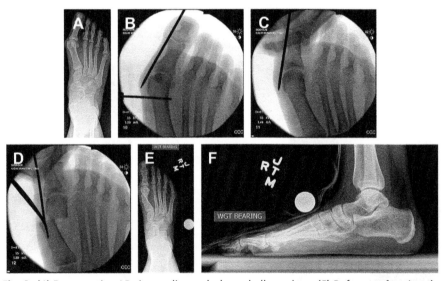

Fig. 6. (*A*) Preoperative AP view radiograph shows hallux valgus. (*B*) Before performing the osteotomy, one can appreciate the laterally deviated sesamoids and the metatarsal head deformity. (*C*) After the osteotomy, the surgeon (N.A.S.) performed a rotation and reduction maneuver to realign the sesamoids. Note that no translation has been performed. (*D*) Capital fragment was translated more than 90% of the diameter of the shaft of the metatarsal while appropriate radiographic alignment of the sesamoid apparatus was maintained. (*E, F*) Postoperative AP (*E*) and lateral (*F*) views showing excellent healing, robust callus formation, and anatomic realignment of the first MPJ. WGT, weight. (*Courtesy of* Rubin Institute for Advanced Orthopedics, Sinai Hospital of Baltimore, Baltimore, MD. Copyright 2018.)

Maintain Relative Stability of the Osteotomy

Bone healing occurs via primary or secondary methods. With minimally invasive correction (first generation), typically no fixation is placed into the capital fragment. The fixation that is used is a single 2.0-mm Steinmann pin from the hallux into the metatarsal medullary canal. The hallux is overcorrected in an adducted position, and the pin buttresses against the capital fragment laterally and the medial flare of the stationary metatarsal medially. The long arm of the pin can extend past the first metatarsal-cuneiform articulation into the medial cuneiform. The metatarsal head is translated laterally up to 90% of the width of the metatarsal. These maneuvers create the necessary soft-tissue tension on the capsular and ligamentous structures about the MPJ. Combined with the medullary pin, the construct imparts relative stability to the osteotomy. Protection in a flat, rigid, surgical shoe provides additional external protection and promotes secondary healing because of the micromotion that occurs during weight bearing. This healing is evidenced by the robust callus that is seen after removal and bone healing (see **Fig. 6**E, F).

Encourage Early Mobilization of the Metatarsophalangeal Joint

This method allows for immediate weight bearing in a protected surgical shoe. The removal of the medullary pin at 4 weeks allows for early ROM exercises and early transition to supportive shoe gear. Unlike open surgery with capsular and ligamentous dissection, this method is all extracapsular, which prevents capsular scarring, intracapsular adhesions, and loss of capsular correction. The ability to perform aggressive ROM and transition to shoe gear sooner has been shown to improve satisfaction.[23]

CASE EXAMPLE: SURGICAL TECHNIQUE IN A DIFFICULT PRESENTATION

A 55-year-old woman with persistent right first MPJ pain presented to the office, reporting pain and discomfort that had been worsening over 4 years. She had tried conservative management by wearing wider shoes and arch supports. The patient had no significant past medical history. She was a smoker but recently had quit her tobacco usage. On physical examination, she presented with a high arched foot and a large dorsal medial prominence. A prominent and inflamed bursa was noted over the dorsal medial prominence. Hypersensitivity of the dorsal digital nerve was noted. Her neurovascular status was intact. She had 5 of 5 muscle strength and 25° of dorsiflexion and plantarflexion. A laterally deviated digit that was reducible to a neutral position was also appreciated.

Radiographic evaluation determined that the hallux valgus angle (HVA), intermetatarsal angle (IMA), and tibial sesamoid position (TSP) were 35°, 16°, and position 4, respectively (**Fig. 7**A). The other notable finding that made this a challenging case was an increased metatarsus adductus angle (MAA) of 28°. The patient underwent a distal metatarsal osteotomy (perspective 1) with the percutaneous method described earlier with placement of internal fixation (third generation) (**Fig. 7**B). An additional percutaneous Akin osteotomy was performed (second generation). The patient presented 2 weeks later at the office after noticing her medullary pin had inadvertently backed out of the metatarsal (**Fig. 7**C). The radiographs showed that her alignment was maintained; therefore, she continued with protected weight-bearing status in the surgical shoe. She transitioned to sturdy sneakers at 4 weeks and went on to heal uneventfully with excellent bony union at 10 weeks (**Fig. 7**D). However, 9 months after surgery, she reported hardware irritation and underwent hardware removal (**Fig. 7**E, F). At her 2.5-year follow-up, the toe had maintained anatomic alignment and she was very satisfied with her clinical outcome.

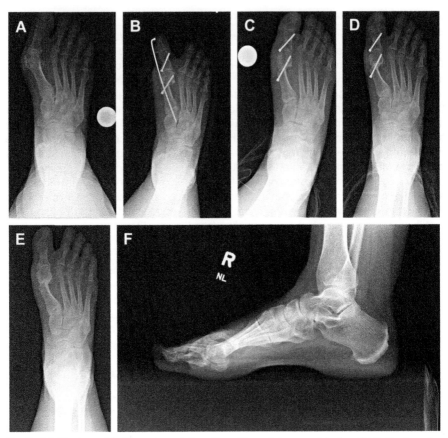

Fig. 7. (*A*) AP view of hallux valgus deformity with metatarsus adductus. (*B*) Patient underwent a percutaneous, minimally invasive bunion correction. (*C*) Patient presented with hardware loosening, and pin was removed. (*D*) Note healing at osteotomy site. However, hardware irritation from screws was noted. (*E, F*) At 2.5-year follow-up, the patient maintained realignment and had excellent ROM with no pain. (*Courtesy of* Rubin Institute for Advanced Orthopedics, Sinai Hospital of Baltimore, Baltimore, MD. Copyright 2018.)

CASE 2: WHEN DEEP INFECTION OCCURS

A 45-year-old woman presented with a progressively worsening bunion deformity that had not responded to conservative management. She started developing transfer metatarsalgia and a dislocation of the second digit (**Fig. 8**A). She was referred by her local podiatrist for surgical management. Her past medical history was significant for hypertension and non–insulin-dependent diabetes mellitus that was well controlled with oral medications and diet. She had previous history of uterine cancer, which had been treated with a hysterectomy. Her hemoglobin A1c was optimized at 6.0%. Clinically, she had a moderate-appearing bunion with pain over the dorsal medial prominence of the first metatarsal. She had 20° of dorsiflexion and plantarflexion of the MPJ. A dorsally dislocated second digit was appreciated with pain and a positive Lachman test. Because of the discomfort in her forefoot, she decided on surgical intervention with a minimally invasive bunion correction, a plantar plate repair of the second MPJ, and digital contracture repair of the second digit.

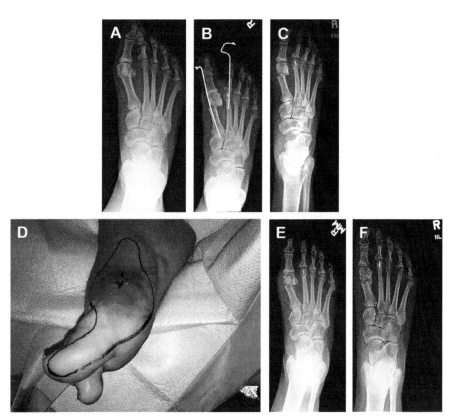

Fig. 8. (A) Preoperative radiograph demonstrating hallux valgus deformity with instability of the second MPJ. (B) Percutaneous bunionectomy with second MPJ plantar plate repair. (C) Radiograph obtained after pin removal. No obvious signs of bony destruction or deep infection were noted. (D) Patient presented to emergency departmet stating she was in pain. Note the intense local infection concerning for a deep infection. (E) Patient presented to the emergency department with increased drainage and radiographic signs of increased lucency, concerning for a deep infection. (F) Radiograph obtained 6 weeks after bunionectomy that was complicated with deep infection. Signs of callus and healing noted. Clinically, the patient was asymptomatic with no pain and had normalization of infection markers after incision and drainage. (*Courtesy of* Rubin Institute for Advanced Orthopedics, Sinai Hospital of Baltimore, Baltimore, MD. Copyright 2018.)

Surgical correction consisted of the hallux valgus deformity, with the surgical technique described earlier (perspective 1), along with a plantar plate repair of the second MPJ (**Fig. 8**B). The patient had an uneventful course during the first 4 weeks after surgery but experienced a fall and injury to her pin site a few days before her second postoperative visit. She had severe pain and an inflamed pin site with ascending redness and drainage. Her incision sites were healed, and the radiographs were negative for any bony destruction or signs of osteomyelitis (**Fig. 8**C). Her pin was removed, and she began orally administered broad-spectrum antibiotics after a culture of the pin site was obtained. Her office cultures revealed a methicillin-sensitive *Staphylococcus aureus* (MSSA) infection. The broad-spectrum antibiotics that were prescribed earlier were sensitive to the cultures; therefore, she continued these antibiotics for 2 weeks. After a brief course, her pain and symptoms resolved. Her weight-bearing status was advanced per the protocol mentioned earlier, and she transitioned to normal shoe gear.

Approximately 3 weeks later, she presented to the emergency department with increased redness, swelling, and a draining wound at the previously healed incision site (**Fig. 8D**). Her radiographs demonstrated lucency and signs of bony destruction (**Fig. 8E**). She was admitted for intravenous antibiotics and underwent evaluation with a indium-111 nuclear scan (she did not undergo evaluation with MRI because she had recent surgery and it may return a false-positive test). Her indium scan was positive for increased uptake and acute osteomyelitis. She was taken to the operating room for incision, drainage, and bone biopsy. Intraoperative findings were positive for signs of a sinus tract to the osteotomy and bony destruction; however, no significant bone loss was appreciated. The previous osteotomy was debrided, and a bone biopsy was sent for cultures and sensitivities. An infectious disease consultation was obtained, and definitive cultures were positive for an MSSA infection. A decision to place a peripheral-inserted central catheter line was made. She began antibiotics for 6 weeks with weekly monitoring of her complete blood count with differential (CBC with diff), erythrocyte sedimentation rate (ESR), and C-reactive protein (CRP). After 6 weeks, her CBC with diff, ESR, and CRP had normalized and the metatarsal started to show signs of radiographic healing (**Fig. 8F**). At her most recent follow-up (6 months), she had not had any recurrence or pain at the osteotomy site and signs of bony consolidation and callus formation were noted. The patient was instructed to follow-up in 6 months or sooner if symptoms recurred.

CASE 3: THERE IS A LEARNING CURVE

A 62-year-old woman had prior flatfoot reconstruction with an adjunctive percutaneous bunionectomy. The patient presented to the office for a second opinion with persistent pain and difficultly with ambulation for many weeks after being told that she had healed after undergoing a reconstructive procedure. She was having severe pain at the first metatarsal osteotomy site and during ambulation. Hypersensitivity was noted along the dorsum and medial aspect of the first metatarsal, and the patient had diffuse lateral column pain. Minimal, well-healed incisions were noted over the first metatarsal and calcaneus. Vascular status was intact, and muscle strength was diminished. The most recent radiographs that were obtained during treatment with the previous surgeon were reviewed, and immediate concerns were raised (**Fig. 9A, B**). New radiographs were obtained that revealed a nonunion/delayed union of the first metatarsal osteotomy and the anterior neck of the calcaneus with persistent subluxation of the calcaneocuboid joint (CCJ). On the lateral view projection, the first metatarsal head/capital fragment was plantarflexed and in malposition (**Fig. 9C, D**). Severe pain with attempted ROM was noted. A decision to return to the operating room was made to correct the malposition of the MPJ, correct the residual hindfoot valgus deformity, and repair the subluxation of the CCJ. The patient underwent a first MPJ fusion, a medial displacement calcaneal osteotomy, and a reduction of the CCJ dislocation. The patient's painful symptoms, after revision, completely resolved. At the 1-year follow-up, the patient had well-healed incisions and complete bony consolidation of the revised surgical sites (**Fig. 9E, F**).

DISCUSSION

Percutaneous or minimally invasive surgical methods are gaining popularity in foot and ankle surgery. The benefits of using a small incisional approach in bunion correction are[15,19,23]

- Minimal bony and soft-tissue disruption
- Decreased operating room time

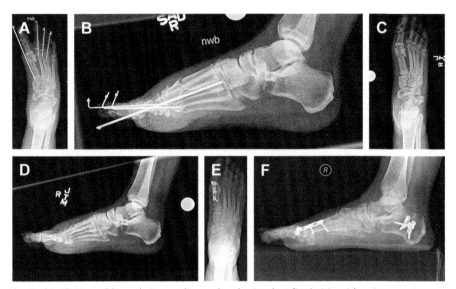

Fig. 9. (*A, B*) AP and lateral view radiographs obtained at final visit with prior treating surgeon. (*C*) AP view radiograph shows nonunion at metatarsal osteotomy site. Additionally, calcaneocuboid joint dislocation (CCJ) is appreciated. (*D*) Lateral view radiograph shows plantarflexed nonunion of the first metatarsal head with dislocated CCJ. (*E*) AP view radiograph obtained 1 year after revision shows a healed first MPJ fusion and correction of the CCJ dislocation. (*F*) Lateral view radiograph shows excellent union of the first MPJ fusion. Note the medial displacement calcaneal osteotomy to correct the residual hindfoot valgus. (*Courtesy of* Rubin Institute for Advanced Orthopedics, Sinai Hospital of Baltimore, Baltimore, MD. Copyright 2018.)

- Earlier weight bearing and rehabilitation
- Increased patient satisfaction
- Decreased cost

A review of the literature reveals that percutaneous bunion correction has been performed more commonly by European and Asian surgeons when compared with North American foot and ankle surgeons.[18] Many procedures have been described to correct hallux valgus through small incisions and have used similar terms, such as *percutaneous*, *minimally invasive*, and *microsurgery*.[18] However, given the variations in technique, Bia and colleagues[18] thought that the concepts in the different methods should not be used interchangeably. They[18] performed a systematic review and redefined these methods as percutaneous forefoot surgery (PFS). Their definition of PFS encompassed hallux valgus correction through a small incision with a burr or saw under fluoroscopic guidance. The goal of the article was to review the current data and provide the best technique for each case. After screening 95 studies, they included 18 studies that met their inclusion criteria. The investigators[18] noted that most studies were case series/observational (level 4) and only 2 were prospective (level 2). They noted that all studies demonstrated reduction and correction of the radiographic and clinical parameters that were compared preoperatively and postoperatively (HVA, IMA, American Orthopedic Foot and Ankle scores).[18] However, the differences in the methods made it difficult to recommend a specific method.

The cases presented in the current article demonstrate common challenges that foot and ankle surgeons will encounter when performing this method of correction.

It has been reported that distal osteotomies tend to have poorer outcomes when performed in patients with metatarsus adductus.[24] Aiyer and colleagues[24] recommended using proximal metatarsal osteotomies or metatarsal-cuneiform fusions with lesser metatarsal osteotomies for correction. However, the investigators successfully demonstrated using this percutaneous method to achieve an excellent correction without adding greater complexity to the correction.

Various complications have also been reported with the diverse methods of minimally invasive corrections.[14,15,18,25,26] These complications can be attributed to the steep learning curve and other preoperative, intraoperative, and postoperative factors.[18,26] The authors of the current article present a case with the most common concern for any operation, which is a superficial or deep infection. Superficial infections are not common and can be managed routinely with orally administered antibiotics.[14,15] Deep infections are even less common and should be treated aggressively, similar to the management for open surgical procedures.[26]

To obtain positive outcomes, Magnan and colleagues[15] stressed strict adherence to the technique described by experienced surgeons. Case number 3 (see **Fig. 9**) accurately demonstrates what can occur if one deviates from these principles. This case had a poor initial outcome even though the surgery was performed by an experienced, fellowship-trained foot and ankle surgeon. The immediate postoperative radiographs demonstrate a lack of surgeon experience with performing percutaneous hallux valgus correction. The percutaneous pin did not maintain good bony apposition distally with the phalanx and was not placed through the medullary canal. It seemed to be engaging only the soft tissue, likely causing the nerve symptoms the patient complained of before revision. The metatarsal head appeared well aligned in the AP view but was severely plantarflexed in the lateral view, which created painful ROM. In this instance, the author (N.A.S.) thought that a definitive first MPJ fusion was the best option for resolution of symptoms, although one could certainly consider an open revision and attempt joint salvage.

The authors have modified the European methods[11,14–16] and have successfully performed these methods in more than 300 feet. The authors are in the process of reporting their outcomes and have observed improvement in preoperative and postoperative radiographic measurements (HVA, TSP, IMA) as reported by others.[11,12,14–16,23] However, the authors agree and reinforce that strict adherence to a specific systematic method is key during the initial phases of learning this powerful method of correction. Slight modification to the slope of the osteotomy, utilization of internal fixation, adjunctive procedures, and double-level corrections can be performed with confidence once the surgeon is comfortable with the methods described earlier.

In conclusion, the authors think the techniques described earlier for minimally invasive hallux valgus correction are equivalent to traditional open procedures and should be considered an excellent alternative for correction of mild, moderate, and severe hallux valgus deformity.

REFERENCES

1. Sim-Fook L, Hodgson AR. A comparison of foot forms among the non-shoe and shoe-wearing Chinese population. J Bone Joint Surg Am 1958;40-A(5):1058–62.
2. Hardy RH, Clapham JC. Observations on hallux valgus: based on a controlled series. J Bone Joint Surg Br 1951;33-B:376–91.
3. Mann RA, Coughlin MJ. Adult hallux valgus. In: Coughlin MJ, Mann RA, editors. Surgery of the foot and ankle, vol. 1, 7th edition. St Louis (MO): Mosby Inc; 1999. p. 150–269.

4. Coughlin MJ, Shurnas PS. Hallux valgus in men. Part II: first ray mobility after bunionectomy and factors associated with hallux valgus deformity. Foot Ankle Int 2003;24(1):73–8.
5. Coughlin MJ, Roger A. Mann Award. Juvenile hallux valgus: etiology and treatment. Foot Ankle Int 1995;16(11):682–97.
6. Trnka H, Hofstaetter SG. Distal chevron osteotomy: perspective 1. In: Easley ME, Wiesel SW, editors. Operative techniques in foot and ankle surgery. Philadelphia: Lippincott Williams & Wilkins; 2011. p. 1–7.
7. Easley ME, Wiesel SW, editors. Operative techniques in foot and ankle surgery. Philadelphia: Lippincott Williams & Wilkins; 2011. p. 8–24.
8. Easley ME, Wiesel SW, editors. Operative techniques in foot and ankle surgery. Philadelphia: Lippincott Williams & Wilkins; 2011. p. 41–83.
9. Scharer BM, DeVries JG. Comparison of chevron and distal oblique osteotomy for bunion correction. J Foot Ankle Surg 2016;55(4):738–42.
10. Schneider W, Aigner N, Pinggera O, et al. Chevron osteotomy in hallux valgus. Ten-year results of 112 cases. J Bone Joint Surg Br 2004;86(7):1016–20.
11. Bösch P, Markowski H, Rannicher V. Technik und erste ergebnisse der subkutanen distalen metatarsale, I osteotomie. Orthopaedische Praxis 1990;26:51–6.
12. Bösch P, Wanke S, Legenstein R. Hallux valgus correction by the method of Bösch: a new technique with a seven-to-ten-year follow-up. Foot Ankle Clin 2000;5(3):485–98.
13. Isham SA. The Reverdin-Isham procedure for the correction of hallux abducto valgus. A distal metatarsal osteotomy procedure. Clin Podiatr Med Surg 1991; 8(1):81–94.
14. Giannini S, Ceccarelli F, Bevoni R, et al. Hallux valgus surgery: the minimally invasive bunion correction (SERI). Tech Foot Ankle Surg 2003;2(1):11–20.
15. Magnan B, Pezzè L, Rossi N, et al. Percutaneous distal metatarsal osteotomy for correction of hallux valgus. J Bone Joint Surg Am 2005;87(6):1191–9.
16. Brogan K, Voller T, Gee C, et al. Third-generation minimally invasive correction of hallux valgus: technique and early outcomes. Int Orthop 2014;38(10):2115–21.
17. Chan CX, Gan JZ, Chong HC, et al. Two year outcomes of minimally invasive hallux valgus surgery. Foot Ankle Surg 2017. [Epub ahead of print].
18. Bia A, Guerra-Pinto F, Pereira BS, et al. Percutaneous osteotomies in hallux valgus: a systematic review. J Foot Ankle Surg 2018;57(1):123–30.
19. Siddiqui NA. A guide to the percutaneous bunionectomy. Podiatry Today 2016; 29(6):32–9.
20. Vernois J, Redfern DJ. Percutaneous surgery for severe hallux valgus. Foot Ankle Clin 2016;21(3):479–93.
21. LaPorta GA, Nasser EM, Mulhern JL, et al. The mechanical axis of the first ray: a radiographic assessment in hallux abducto valgus evaluation. J Foot Ankle Surg 2016;55(1):28–34.
22. Siddiqui NA, Sharma P, Fink J, et al. Mechanical axis method to determine first intermetatarsal angle and tibial sesamoid position. Poster presented at the Annual Meeting of the American College of Foot and Ankle Surgeons. Nashville, TN, March, 2018.
23. Radwan YA, Mansour AM. Percutaneous distal metatarsal osteotomy versus distal chevron osteotomy for correction of mild-to-moderate hallux valgus deformity. Arch Orthop Trauma Surg 2012;132(11):1539–46.
24. Aiyer A, Shub J, Shariff R, et al. Radiographic recurrence of deformity after hallux valgus surgery in patients with metatarsus adductus. Foot Ankle Int 2016;37(2): 165–71.

25. Kadakia AR, Smerek JP, Myerson MS. Radiographic results after percutaneous distal metatarsal osteotomy for correction of hallux valgus deformity. Foot Ankle Int 2007;28(3):355–60.
26. Yanez Arauz JM. Treatment of minimally invasive hallux valgus surgery complications. Tech Foot Ankle 2017;16:11–9.

3D Printed Total Talar Replacement

A Promising Treatment Option for Advanced Arthritis, Avascular Osteonecrosis, and Osteomyelitis of the Ankle

Helen Shnol, DPM*, Guido A. LaPorta, DPM, MS

KEYWORDS

- 3D printed talus • Avascular necrosis • Tarsal osteomyelitis
- Total talus replacement • End-stage ankle arthritis

KEY POINTS

- End-stage arthritis in younger individuals has few functional options for reconstruction.
- A 3D printed talus provides an anatomically accurate replacement for the compromised ankle.
- Talar replacement procedures also address arthritic deformities in adjacent tarsal joints.
- Total talar replacement may provide the best option for younger patients with end-stage ankle pathology.

INTRODUCTION

Advanced ankle arthritis (osteoarthritis [OA]), avascular osteonecrosis (AVN), and osteomyelitis (OM) of the ankle remain a surgical challenge in the foot and ankle arena with limited treatment options.[1–5] The tibia, fibula, and the talus form a stable ring-like construct to maintain stability of the ankle joint; however, it is the talus' role in mediating the fibro-osseous connection between the foot and ankle that potentiates locomotion and guides the sagittal motion of the lower extremity.[6] Multiple medical comorbidities including but not limited to autoimmune disease, trauma, avascular necrosis,[1,2,7,8] or other idiopathic causes contribute to total loss of the talus.[3–5,9–11] Furthermore, collapse of the talar body as a complication of total ankle arthroplasty,[12] talectomy in infection and septic talus necrosis,[13] or severe bone defects caused by

Disclosure Statement: None.
Department of Graduate Medical Education and Podiatric Surgery, Our Lady of Lourdes Memorial Hospital, 169 Riverside Drive, Binghamton, NY 13905, USA
* Corresponding author.
E-mail address: helen.shnol@gmail.com

Clin Podiatr Med Surg 35 (2018) 403–422
https://doi.org/10.1016/j.cpm.2018.06.002
0891-8422/18/© 2018 Elsevier Inc. All rights reserved.

tumor resection[14] may result in the need for total talar replacement (TTR), especially in younger and active patients. Ankle arthrodesis, with or without an allograft or the complete rearfoot, and tibiocalcaneal fusion after talectomy can produce severe disability of the ankle and the foot.[14] Total ankle replacement (TAR) is another viable option for treatment of end-stage AO in appropriate patient population; however, risks of subsidence and loosening of the talar component are still prevalent.[14–16]

Implantation of a custom made talar body[17–20] or TTR[12,21–24] has shown encouraging results. Harnroongroj and Vanadurongwan[17] was the first to document outcomes of 16 patients treated by first-generation talar body prosthesis in 1997. Eight out of nine patients, who were evaluated 11 to 15 years postoperatively, had a satisfactory result. In 2014, Harnroongroj and Harnroongroj[18] published outcomes in a study with the longest follow-up period of 10 to 36 years; 28 of the 33 talar body prosthesis were still in place and five had failed before 5 years. In 1999, Tanaka and colleagues[25] designed talar body prosthesis to preserve ankle motion in patients with aseptic necrosis, followed by several subsequent prosthesis design revisions to improve outcomes after prosthesis implantation.[18] Taniguchi and colleagues[20] explored two types of talar body prosthesis. The first-generation used a peg for the neck of the talus and second-generation removed the peg. Despite acceptable results in eight of 14 patients treated with the latter implant, the author recommended TTR after a mean follow-up period of 98 months. In 2005, Taniguchi and colleagues[23] reported excellent primary outcomes of postoperative function and pain in 55 patients with osteonecrosis of the talus treated with prosthetic TTR.

Talar body and TTR use further expanded to young and more active patients. In 2004, Magnan and colleagues[19] first reported use of talar body prosthesis combined with standard Scandinavian total ankle replacement (STAR) system in a professional 45-year-old male skier and rock-climber who sustained open talar dislocation and medial malleolar fracture. Stevens and colleagues[24] first reported TTR after traumatic open talar extrusion in a 14-year-old patient in 2007. Other investigators incorporated and modified TAR to address talar pathologies.

Lampert[14] had successfully combined TTR with HINTEGRA (Newdeal, Lyon, France/Integra, Plainsboro, NJ) in three patients with talar bone tumor, AVN, and TAR complication. Ketz and colleagues[16] noted an increase in total ankle joint motion from 21.3°± 14° to 32.2° ± 11° in 33 patients with rearfoot arthritis and revision of failed TAR. All patients were treated with total ankle arthroplasties using custom long-stemmed talar components. Giannini and colleagues[26] reported the first custom-made total talonavicular replacement in a professional rock climber after a complex talar and navicular fracture. At 30-month follow-up,[27] full body gait analysis and three-dimensional (3D) joint kinematics showed good restoration of rotation and no evidence of kinematic changes in the neighboring joints of the foot. Therefore, use of TTR with or without tibial component modifications provides another viable source to address ankle and hindfoot pathologies.

This article discusses functional paradoxes that make the ankle joint a unique and fascinating articulation and introduces TTR, a surgical treatment option that embraces talus' distinct role within an ankle joint. TTR is outlined with presentation of most recent research data to replace the talar body[1,2,10,19,20] and the complete talus,[12,21–24] in addition to a review of pertinent talar anatomy, biomechanical features, indications for TTR, types of prosthesis, and procedure overview.

ANATOMIC AND BIOMECHANICAL CONSIDERATIONS

The ankle joint is a rolling joint that gains most of its stability from osseous and ligamentous structures. The static stabilization of the ankle is maintained by the medial ligamentous structures, interosseous membrane, tibiofibular, lateral collateral ligaments, and tendinous structures. In addition to these structures, the talus also provides structure but is unique because of the presence of multiple of strong ligamentous structures, while being devoid of any tendon or muscular attachments. The talus articulates with the tibial plafond, medial and lateral malleoli, the calcaneus, and navicular.[23,28,29] Congruence of distal articular surface of the tibia, fibula, and trochlear surface of the talus aids in even distribution of weight-bearing forces on the joint.[6,30,31] Various mechanical, biochemical, and anatomic peculiarities of the ankle account for its apparent resilience to aging and trauma.

Unlike the hip or the knee, the ankle is efficient at dispersing locomotion despite its minimal cartilaginous padding. The ankle joint also has a significantly smaller surface area than the hip or knee, yet it withstands five times the body weight when walking and up to 13 times the body weight when running.[30–34] The ankle has a thin uniform cartilage profile, measuring 1 to 1.7 mm, with much higher compressive modulus making it less elastic and more prone to subchondral changes in the event of joint incongruity.[30,31,34–36] Although ankle cartilage does not decrease in tensile strength with age,[30,31,34,35,37] it may develop fissures attributable to overuse. However, this condition does not progress to OA as it would in the knee or hip.[30,31,34,35] Ankle chondrocytes have decreased sensitivity to inflammatory proteins, such as interleukin-1 and matrix metalloproteinases, in particular matrix metalloproteinase-8, which is usually elevated in OA.[6,30,31,34,35] As a result, the ankle joint is unlikely to succumb to damage by inflammatory changes alone, unless there is a disruption of talar anatomy.

Many factors, including cartilage thickness, mechanical, and metabolic factors predispose the ankle to post-traumatic arthritis, with ankle OA having a strong predilection among females.[30,31,34,35] The combination of large cartilaginous area covering at least 56.9% of the total talar dome surface[38] and a precarious blood supply make the talar body more susceptible to traumatic or idiopathic osteonecrosis. Predictably, the talus is found in the top three anatomic locations of idiopathic necrosis, preceded by the femoral head and femoral condyle, respectively.[39]

The head, neck, and body of the talus are supplied by the dorsalis pedis, the artery of the sinus tarsi, and the artery of the tarsal canal. The rich anastomotic network around the talar head and neck regions is formed by the superior neck vessels, including dorsalis pedis and the artery of the sinus tarsi. Gadolinium-enhanced MRI study has confirmed sources of arterial blood supply and described a new direct branch to the medial aspect of the talar neck from the posterior tibial artery. This newly identified branch was consistently noted to be lacerated following a standard anteromedial surgical approach to the talar neck in 9 of 12 cadaver specimens. An anterolateral approach to the talus did not seem to disrupt any major blood supply. Overall contribution of blood supply to the talus from the posterior tibial, anterior tibial, and peroneal arteries was recorded at 47%, 36.2%, and 16.9%, respectively.[40]

Another study on the microvascular network of the talus identified the highest amount and density of nutritive foramina in the sulcus tali.[38] Osteonecrosis of talar head and neck is extremely rare, unlike that of the talar body. Talar body injuries have a poor healing prognosis because of the vulnerable position of the artery of the tarsal canal as it courses along the inferior aspect of the talus from the opening of the tarsal canal to sinus tarsi and superior calcaneus. The degree of displacement of the body increases osteonecrosis rates up to 100% based on Hawkins classifications.[23,29,38,40–42]

The role of the talus within the ankle joint is of particular interest because it mediates the sagittal movement of the leg and foot during gait.[6,43] Parlous blood supply and overall anatomy of the talus predisposes the bone to higher risk of osteonecrosis following traumatic injuries.[28] Knowledge of the biomechanical and anatomic considerations of patients with OA, AVN, or OM is of utmost importance to create the best treatment plan.

INDICATIONS FOR TOTAL TALAR PROSTHESIS USE
Degenerative Joint Disease of the Ankle

The tibiotalar joint is more resistant to development of primary OA than hips or knees.[44] Primary ankle OA is estimated to occur in 1% of the population[6,31] with up to 78% of reports resulting from trauma.[30,31,34,45,46] The remaining 22% results from neuroarthropathy, rheumatoid arthritis,[12] hemochromatosis, and inflammatory arthropathies.[30,31,34,45] Sitting cross-legged or with legs tucked under can also contribute to arthritic changes in the ankle in up to 20% of patients.[47,48]

Most arthritis seen in the ankle is caused by post-traumatic changes, especially among active young adults. This post-traumatic arthritis is typically attributed to the severity of the initial injury and reduction quality of the original fractures.[30,31,45] Asymmetric wear and progression of degeneration stems from major ankle trauma, such as tibial plafond fractures, talar dome or neck fractures, osteochondral defects, large posterior malleolar fractures with displacement, 40% of bimalleolar, and up to 71% of trimalleolar fractures.[30,31,47–52] Fourteen percent of posttraumatic arthritis results from ankle fractures with up to 33% of those cases having Wb C fractures.[30,50] Fibular shortening and malrotation (or a combination of the two) can lead to talar tilt or ankle instability depending on the severity of the deformity.[30,31,44]

Degenerative changes can also stem from distal tibial osteonecrosis, intra-articular changes related to chronic cavovarus with or without lateral ankle instability, flatfoot deformity, hindfoot varus, and peroneal tendon dysfunction.[53] Development of OA increases with the extent of the chondral injury,[52] where as little as 1-mm lateral shift of the tibiotalar articulation causes reduction in the contact area, increases pressure, and thus disrupts the congruity of the joint.[30,54] Ankle OA has a tremendous impact on mobility and activities of daily living in younger and active patients. In the study of 406 patients, 78% of patients younger than 60 years old were most commonly affected by OA. Besides reduced walking speed and shorter stride, most documented sequela of OA is the decreased range of motion (ROM) of the ankle, especially in the sagittal plane.

Limited dorsiflexion and plantar flexion translate to an increased stress on the hip, knee, and subtalar joints as compensatory mechanisms. Therefore, ankle fusion should be offered as a last surgical option for treatment of OA. Other options, such as TAR and TTR, mimic physiologic ankle joint ROM and its biomechanics. However, unlike the TAR, TTR does not present the same challenges of implant loosening, subsidence, or failure and is the superior treatment.

Avascular Osteonecrosis

Avascular necrosis of the talus poses a significant problem because collapse of the talar dome leads to degenerative changes, pain, and disability of the ankle and subtalar joints. Top three causes of AVN are trauma; medications; and autoimmune diseases, such as lupus or sickle cell disease. Up to 75% of cases of AVN are traumatically induced in association with talar neck and body fractures.[42] Literature search for talar trauma has strong evidence to support use of TTR as a promising treatment to address post-traumatic osteonecrosis. Although there are many published treatments for posttraumatic AVN of the talus, critical outcome studies are still lacking.[55]

Current treatment options of talar AVN depend on degree of displacement of the body and distribution of the AVN within the talar dome, based on the Hawkins classification.[42] The higher this stage, the more involved the surgical intervention is to remove the necrotic bone. The greater the bone loss, the more plates, intramedullary nails, or external fixators are used to restore ankle position and stability. If only the ankle joint is involved, tibiotalar fusion with or without bone graft is often considered. However, when talar body is osteonecrotic or sustained traumatic comminuted talar body fracture, Blair[56] first recommended surgical excision of the talar body and translation of the anterior tibial cortex onto the talar neck to create an onlay graft. Many authors have modified the Blair technique to fuse the tibiotalar joint and to treat AVN simultaneously, but results have been mixed and depended on the degree of bone loss. Although modified Blair procedure may be a good surgical choice for some patients, tibiotalocalcaneal arthrodesis provides a better outcome in advanced cases of AVN.[57]

Regardless of the procedure, there are risks and complications associated with any surgery. Major complications associated with these types of procedures include loss of limb function, limb length discrepancy,[58] and risk of pseudarthrosis.[59] Although use of a bone allograft, such as femoral head, can compensate for the bone void, use of anatomically correct implant is a more viable option to maintain leg length and joint function.[23]

Multiple authors strongly advocate for the use of TTR in patients with idiopathic and post-traumatic arthritis.[17,18,20,21,23] Prosthetic total talar implant is a useful procedure for patients with osteonecrosis of the talus because the favorable congruency of the custom-made implant with the adjacent joints produces stability and maintains ankle function.[23]

Osteomyelitis

OM, or inflammation of the bone caused by an infecting microorganism, remains one of the most challenging clinical problems among providers. Multispecialty involvement of the vascular surgery, foot and ankle surgery, and infectious disease services reduces mortality from OM. Regardless of its cause or staging, discussion of treatment with antibiotics versus cure with surgical intervention is warranted between the provider and their patient. In the presence of systemic response to OM, resection of the affected bone remains the gold standard of treatment. Resection of nonessential bones in the foot and ankle, such as metatarsals, tarsals, partial calcaneus, and fibula, is done with satisfactory retention of the function.[60] However, what happens when there is an assault to an "essential" bone, such as the talus in instances of bone inflammation or trauma? What if OM of the talus can be treated the same way as an extruded talus?

Total talectomy has been used most commonly to treat children with congenital deformities, such as severe clubfoot deformity, arthrogryposis multiplex congenita, myelomeningocele, tuberculosis, and tumors. In adults, it has been used in salvage procedures that involve trauma, nonunion of ankle fusions, failed total ankle arthroplasty, inflammatory arthropathy, neuroarthropathy, failed talar prosthesis, failed pantalar fusions, adult neglected clubfoot, post-traumatic avascular necrosis talus, and deformities that are caused by sciatic nerve palsy and compartment syndrome.[60,61] Blair[56] described the first tibiocalcaneal fusion for fracture-dislocations with AVN of the talar body.[57-59] Blair advocated for tibiocalcaneal fusion based on aesthetics of the foot, realignment of the foot and leg and maintenance of the limb length, distribution of weight-bearing surface across the joint surface, and retention of some sagittal motion.[56] The Blair fusion may be used to achieve an ankle arthrodesis in the presence of AVN or absent talar body. Despite using up to 2 cm of tibial cortical graft to maintain overall limb length, there is still pseudarthrosis rate of 28%.[56–59]

Several prior studies showed a strong penchant for primary fusion of the ankle following talus extrusion, based on the premise that the development of infection and AVN are inevitable and lead to uniformly poor outcomes.[62–64] Detenbeck and Kelly[64] lobbied against primary fusion because of 38% of patients with reported infection within first month of the injury that affected functional and clinical outcomes. Canale and Kelly[65] reported rates of AVN up to 90%[48] in traumatic injuries of the talus. Based on high infection and high AVN rates, the aforementioned authors also concluded that reimplantation of the extruded talus was contraindicated. Therefore, infection risk stratification is an important consideration before reimplantation of the native talus or placing an implant. In addition, prosthesis or reimplantation in case of talar extrusion offers many advantages comparable with arthrodesis, such as preserving ankle joint biomechanics with retained joint space height and bone stock.[28] Such procedures as total talectomy can be used to prepare the ankle joint space to eradicate the source of OM and prepare the ankle joint for a talar implant.

Reported OM of the talus following open 3C Gustilo-Anderson fracture had good outcome using primary limb shortening with a talectomy, tibiocalcaneal arthrodesis using external fixation, and a combination of vancomycin-loaded calcium sulfate and intravenous antibiotics.[62"] Burston and colleagues[28] reported fair outcome in a patient with completely extruded talus, who underwent reimplantation of the talus followed by subtalar and talonavicular joints fusion. The patient was able to return to preinjury activities, including skiing and walking, despite eventual finding of AVN of the talar dome.

Some authors have reported encouraging findings with reimplantation, which suggest that a satisfactory patient outcome is possible with this line of management.[28] Brewster and Maffulli[66] presented two cases of talar injuries where all soft tissue attachments were destroyed and, in both cases, the tali were managed with reimplantation without apparent development of infection, and only one of the cases advanced to talus AVN, which was observed at 6 weeks postoperative. Interestingly, after 2 years of follow-up, the radiographic evidence of talus AVN had resolved.

Additionally, Assal and Stern[9] reported a case of left total talar extrusion treated by means of reimplantation without the use of internal fixation. After more than 5 years of follow-up, the authors reported an excellent outcome without infection or AVN. Moreover, that patient was able to ambulate for up to 2 hours, ride a bicycle, and ski with only minor pain.[9]

In the absence of deep infection, development of AVN does not necessarily lead to an unfavorable outcome. Salvaging the talus through talectomy and implant placement, in the absence of infection or gross contamination, therefore seems to be a reasonable consideration for the treatment of talar trauma or OM of the talus versus arthrodesis with or without the interpositional graft, such as femoral head.[28]

Arthrodesis or talectomy for the treatment of AVN of the talus or a severe crush fracture of the body of the talus often produces a disability of the ankle and the foot.[17] Therefore, a prosthesis designed to replace the body of the talus and to preserve the function of the ankle and the foot was developed. The prosthesis has a superior curved surface, and the medial and lateral surfaces are inclined for articulation with the tibia and the fibula. The inferior aspect has a concave curved surface at the posterior aspect of the prosthesis to serve as the posterior facet for articulation with the posterior facet of the calcaneus, and there is a convex curved surface at the anterior aspect of the prosthesis for articulation with the middle facet of the calcaneus. The neck and the head of the talus are preserved to allow insertion of the prosthetic stem into bone.

PROSTHESIS TYPES AND SURGICAL APPROACH

Construction of each prosthesis starts with measurement of the contralateral talus on radiographs of the ankle, MRI, and/or computed tomography (CT) scans.[17,20–23,67] Anteroposterior and lateral views of the ankle are collected to record a first set of measurements of the talar height, length, and width. The CT images are then collected at 2-mm intervals in the axial and sagittal planes to create a 3D model, the implant's first prototype. A stereolithographic model is casted, and from that prosthesis is produced.[17]

Talar dome of the implant is defined by its superior, medial, lateral, and posterior surfaces, all of which are adjusted to match the calculated measurements. Convex surface and posterior aspect of the talar dome are adjusted to ensure congruence with the tibia. The concave outline of the inferior surface of the implant is refined to complement the posterior facet of the calcaneus so the anterior inferior surface of the implant corresponds with the middle facet of the calcaneus. Talar body prosthesis has either entirely convex or transverse anterior surface to recreate articulation with the navicular or neck of the talus, respectively. Multiple templates are used to confirm the thickness and length of the talar body and the width of the posterior facet of the talus when the final shaping of the prosthesis has been completed. These prostheses require up to 4 to 6 weeks to produce. Type of surgical approach is important to reduce rehabilitation morbidity on the patient. In addition, type of material to make an artificial talus is key to match the bone's biologic affinity; therefore, medical-grade stainless steel, alumina ceramic, and cobalt chrome are most commonly used. Yoshinaga[68] reported that alumina ceramic has less wear than 316L stainless steel.

Various studies support the use of talar body implant (**Table 1**) with favorable results. In 1997, Harnroongroj and Vanadurongwan[17] used the transmalleolar approach to implant talar body prosthesis made of stainless steel in patients with avascular necrosis or severe crush fractures. A total of 8 out of 14 patients had a satisfactory result after 11 years of follow-up. One patient underwent revision of the implant because of anterior and inferior subsidence into the talar neck. Between 1999 and 2006, Taniguchi and colleagues[20] treated aseptic necrosis of the talus with first- and second-generation alumina ceramic prosthesis via lateral transmalleolar and anterior approach, respectively. The major difference between the two types of models correlated with a presence of a peg to affix to the head and neck of the talus, as seen in first-generation implant. Six out of eight patients had excellent to fair outcomes with the latter type of prosthesis; however, loosening around the peg was noted in all eight patients. A second version of the prosthesis without fixation to the neck of the talus had excellent to good results in 8 out of 14 patients. Following initially encouraging data from first- and second-generation results, the authors could not recommend the use of talar body prosthesis and endorsed total talar prosthesis instead.

Literature search results also highlight the benefits of the TTR (see **Table 1**), such as restoration of ankle joint function and pain relief in patients with osteonecrosis. Taniguchi and colleagues[23] investigated outcomes of TTR in patients with talar osteonecrosis in 55 ankles from 2005 to 2012. Anterior approach allowed to perform total talectomy and to substitute the void with alumina ceramic implant by simple traction of the foot. No further malleolar osteotomies or ligamentous repairs were required. Ankle instability evaluation via talar tilt angle in inversion and eversion was noted to be negative with angle values to be within normal limits. There was no stress osseous reaction in the tibia, navicular, and calcaneus on lateral radiographs of the ankle. Similar findings were noted in a patient treated with third-

Table 1
Talus prosthesis

Study	Indication	Prosthesis Type	Material	Surgical Approach	Outcomes
Harnroonngroj & Vanadurongwan,[17] 1997	AVN (N = 12), crush injury (N = 4)	Talar body	316L stainless steel	Transmedial malleolar, Posteriormedial ankle	• Satisfactory at 10 y F/U in N = 6 • Satisfactory at 11–15 y F/U in N = 9, 1 out of 9 had revision of the prosthesis • 1 out of N = 16 removed prosthesis and chose tibiotalar arthrodesis
Magnan,[19] 2004	Open total talar dislocation with loss of medial mallelous and deltoid ligament (N = 1)	Total talus using STAR talar hemiprosthesis with custom tibial component with a medial-retaining flange	316L stainless steel	Anteromedial ankle	28 mo F/U results: • Ankle ROM: 5° of DF, 30° of PF • AOFAS ankle-RF: 92 /100 points • RF varus due to poor fit
Stevens,[24] 2007	Open talar extrusion (N = 1)	Total talus	Cobalt-chrome	Anterior ankle	4 y F/U: • DF: 10° (intra-op) to 4° (post-op) • PF: 50° (intra-op) to 20° (post-op)
Taniguchi,[20] 2012	Idiopathic and traumatic AVN N = 22	Talar body with and without neck/head peg, first and second generations respectively	Ceramic	1st gen – Lateral transmalleolar 2nd gen – Anterior ankle	First gen implant 21–174 mo F/U: • 2 out of N = 8 revised • Mean AOFAS: 46.6 to 80/100 • XR - loosening and talar head necrosis in all patients one year post-op Second gen implant 18–118 mo F/U: • 4 out of N = 14 revised • Mean AOFAS: 50.4 to 81.1/100 • Migration of the implant in ½ of the patients • XR – sclerotic changes in tibia or the calcaneus in N = 12
Angthong,[22] 2014	Traumatic AVN N = 4	Total talus	316L stainless steel	Anterior ankle	4.6–10.6 mo F/U: • TTR (N = 1), HINTEGRA TAR (N = 3) • In both groups: ○ Pre-/postop DF: $-1.3 \pm 2.5°/2.5 \pm 2.1°$ ○ Mean PF: 4.3 ± 3.0 to $24.0 \pm 10.8°$ ($P = .03$) ○ Mean ankle ROM: $3.0 \pm 2.4°$ to $26.5 \pm 9.0°$ ($P = .009$)

Harnroongroj & Harnroongro,[18] 2014	AVN (N = 23), comminuted fracture (N = 8), and talar body tumor (N = 2)	Talar body	316L stainless steel	Medial transmalleolar	10–36 y F/U (N = 28) • N = 26 with plantigrade foot, no ankle-RF instability, deformity ○ Median DF: 5° to 0° ○ Mean PF: 32° to 25° (P = .022)
Taniguchi,[23] 2015	AVN N = 55	Total talus	Aluminum	Anterior ankle	24–96 mo F/U: • Total JSSF (in points) 43.1 ± 17.0 to 89.4 ± 8.4 • AOS (in points) Pain: 6.1 to 2.0 ○ Mean DF: 0.5° ± 3.7° to 5.4° ± 4.9° ○ Mean PF: 43.7° ± 8.3° to 32.0° ± 8.9°
Ando,[21] 2016	Idiopathic AVN (N = 1)	Total talus	Aluminum-ceramic	Anterior ankle	F/U at 2 y: ○ Ankle ROM: 20° DF and 40° PF
Regauer,[10] 2017	Traumatic AVN in one cadaveric leg	Total talus: custom hemiprosthesis with tibial component of STAR and eyelets for ATFL, Deltoid, IOTL	316L stainless steel	Anterior ankle	Ankle ROM: • Maximum DF 22° • Maximum PF 28° Varus, valgus, or sagittal stress with 150N: • Maximum anterior talar migration: 6 mm • Maximum varus tilt 3° • Maximum valgus tilt 2°
Ketz,[16] 2012	Stage IV PTTD (N = 6) Failed TAR (N = 13) Ankle and RF OA (N = 13)	Agility long-stemmed talar prosthesis		Anterior ankle	52–66 mo F/U: • Mean DF: 1.4° ± 7° to 6.4° ± 6° (P<.05) • Mean PF: 25.5° ± 12° to 25.8° ± 10° (P = .26) • Total ankle ROM: 21.3° to 32.2° AOFAS: 41 ± 16 to 68 ± 12 (P<.05)

Abbreviations: AOFAS, American Orthopaedic Foot and Ankle Society ankle/hindfoot score; AOS, Ankle osteoarthritis scale; ATFL, anterior talofibular ligament; AVN, Avascular necrosis; DF, Dorsiflexion; F/U, Follow – up; IOTL, interosseous tibial ligament; JSSF, Japanese Society for Surgery of the Foot ankle-hindfoot scale; OA, Osteoarthritis; PF, Plantarflexion; PTTD, Posterior tibial tendon dysfunction; RF, Rearfoot/Hindfoot; ROM, Range of motion; TAR, Total ankle replacement; TTR, Total talar replacement; XR, X-ray.

generation aluminum ceramic total talar implant for idiopathic AVN of the talus.[21] At 2-year follow-up, patient had 20° dorsiflexion, 40° plantarflexion, American Orthopedic Foot and Ankle Society (AOFAS) score of 90, and no evidence of subsidence or reactive stress reactions in adjacent articulations. Angthong[22] treated four patients with post-traumatic AO or talar loss with either Hintegra TAR (N = 3) or a custom total talar prosthesis (N = 1). In a patient with total implant group, visual analog scale foot and ankle (VAS-FA) score increased from 6.0 to 57.5, the Short Form-36 (SF-36) score increased from 19.3 to 73.7, the dorsiflexion increased from 0° to 5°, the plantar flexion increased from 0° to 16°, and the total ankle motion increased from 0° to 21°. The preoperative and postoperative inversion were 0° and 10°, and the eversion were 0° and 13°. TAR group also responded favorable with increase in mean VAS-FA scores from 51.5 ± 15.6 to 85.7 ± 4.7 (P = .032), and mean SF-36 scores increased from 65.2 ± 13.3 to 99.3 ± 1.2 (P = .055). Although there were no statistically significant changes in mean dorsiflexion, plantarflexion, and total ankle motion measurements, both TAR and total talar implant groups proved to be viable treatment options at short-term follow-up.

Other talar implants (see **Table 1**) incorporate either tibial or talar components of TAR systems, especially in patients with large bone defects or OA changes of the immediate neighboring joints. Lampert[14] created a custom-made talus combined with the Hintegra TAR to treat three patients with a tumor, large areas of osteolysis in TAR, and post-traumatic talus body necrosis. The custom-made talus and TAR combination is a practical alternative to a tibiocalcaneal arthrodesis in selected cases with massive defects of the talus. Regauer and coworkers[10] designed and implanted custom made hemiprosthesis using anatomic principles of STAR with additional eyelets for fixation of artificial ligaments, such as anterior tibiofibular ligament, deltoid, interosseous talocalcaneal ligaments, with FiberTape Internal Brace (Arthrex, Naples, FL) technique. Biarticular hemiprosthesis was used with tibial component of STAR TAR system if there was damage to the tibial plafond. Triarticular hemiprosthesis is used in ankle joint with intact articular surfaces. The implant was constructed based on CT and MRI images in a single cadaver leg of a 36-year-old man. No malleolar osteotomies were needed in this instance, and the implant was successfully incorporated via anterior ankle approach.

The allure of the 3D printed talus lies within its anatomic replica and various options to customize the implant. The role of the talus is undoubtedly unique based on its biomechanical and anatomic properties within an ankle joint and during gait. Just as the native talus communicates with contiguous structures via ligaments yet remains vacant of muscular and tendinous attachments, the custom printed bone can meet the same anatomic requirements. Many talar models can be adjusted to incorporate fixation portals for subtalar joint fusion or lateral ankle instability correction with an internal brace. However, the 3D printed talus' undoubted advantage is recreation of the joint congruence to evenly distribute the force and eliminate the source of ankle joint pain.

PROCEDURE HIGHLIGHTS

The patient is prepared and draped in usual aseptic manner, a pneumatic thigh tourniquet was inflated to 325 mm the lower extremity. Attention is directed to the anterior aspect of the ankle where the tibialis anterior and extensor hallucis longus are superficially identified. A 10- to 12-cm midline skin incision is made and carried distally to the level of the talonavicular joint. The incision is deepened through the subcutaneous tissue to the level of the extensor retinaculum. Special care is taken to preserve and retract all neurovascular structures. Deep dissection is performed between the tibialis anterior and extensor hallucis longus tendons down to the level of the ankle joint. The ankle joint capsule is identified, incised and dissected medially and laterally to allow full exposure of the ankle joint and the talus (**Fig. 1**).

The talonavicular joint is identified and mobilized. The microsagittal saw is used to resect the talus, which is removed in multiple pieces until complete visualization of the dorsal calcaneus, subtalar joint, and the tibial plafond is accomplished (**Fig. 2**).

The custom-made total talus implant is placed into the ankle joint. Using a femoral head impactor, the implant is placed into the ankle joint and talonavicular joint (**Fig. 3**). Place the ankle joint through a ROM and note any impingement. Any areas of impingement, specifically in the medial and lateral gutters, need to be addressed at this time. The ankle joint capsule is repaired, followed by subcutaneous tissue and skin closure. A gastrocnemius recession or tendoachilles lengthening is performed as clinically needed. The patient remain nonweightbearing for 2 weeks followed by 4 weeks of protected weightbearing. Strenuous activity is restricted for 4 to 6 months depending on patient tolerance.

HOW TO MEASURE OUTCOMES

Outcome measurement is important to document the efficacy of medical treatments and surgical intervention in patients with lower extremity complaints. Literature

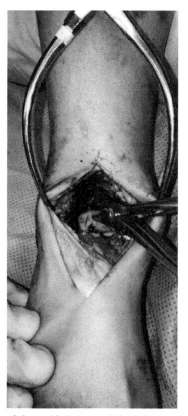

Fig. 1. Allow full exposure of the ankle joint and the talus.

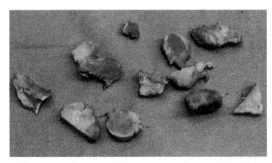

Fig. 2. Resect the talus until there is complete visualization of the calcaneus and tibia.

documenting a standardized method to measure ankle joint ROM after TAR or total talar prosthesis implantation is scant and inconsistent. Most of the available measurements are a result of combination of clinical examination, imaging, and various rating systems. There are outcome measures designed for TAR; however, none are yet available for TTR.[69]

Other than comparing outcomes with improvements in ankle dorsiflexion up to 20° and plantarflexion up to 50°, there is no standardized approach to measure ROM after total ankle arthroplasty.[69] Total talus implant should show advancement in total ankle motion and with essential daily activities. In addition to analysis of the deformity on

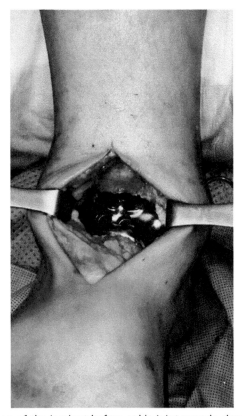

Fig. 3. Inspect position of the implant before ankle joint capsule closure.

standard anteroposterior, lateral, and Saltzman ankle films, consider an in-depth evaluation of proximal limb to check for the center of rotation of angulation to maximize the longevity of the implant.

The lateral distal tibial angle ranges from 86° to 92° between the anatomic axis of the tibia and ankle joint orientation line and measures deformity in the frontal plane. Increase or decrease in lateral distal tibial angle corresponds with valgus or varus distal tibia deformity, respectively. Subtalar joint plays a major role in deformity compensation and can tolerate up to 30° of inversion. Any deformity greater that requires more than 30° of inversion seeks compensation through adjacent joints, and therefore results in pathology of neighboring joints.[70]

The anterior distal tibial angle ranges from 78° to 82° between the mechanical axis of the tibia and ankle joint orientation line and identifies deformity in the sagittal plane, such as recurvatum or procurvatum. Recurvatum deformity is less likely to require correction because the ankle can compensate via larger plantarflexory ROM of up to 50° than 20° of dorsiflexion. The ankle is less tolerant of the procurvatum force and therefore found to be more symptomatic, often requiring surgical correction.[70]

Coetzee and Castro[69] observed statistically significant improvement in tibiotalar ROM by 5° based on serial preoperative and postoperative radiographs in 50 Agility (DePuy Orthopedics, Warsaw, IN) TARs. Preoperative ROM proved to be the main factor determining the eventual postoperative ROM. The numbers were not large enough to make specific statistical conclusions, but a trend emerged. Patients with little motion preoperatively had a trend to a slight increase in ROM postoperatively. Patients with a good ROM preoperatively maintain or might lose some motion. If the patient begins with reasonable motion, approximately the same motion should be maintained. Ankle replacement surgery does not increase ROM dramatically, but with the reduction in pain, the patient seems to be able to use the ROM more effectively. Serial lateral radiographs of ankles in weightbearing position were taken preoperatively and at 1-year postoperative follow-up. Ankle, midfoot, and combined ROM also were documented during the same appointments. Initial tibiotalar ROM of 18.5° improved to 23.4°, and combined midfoot and ankle motion increased from 25.1° to 31.3° after Agility ankle arthroplasty.

Clinical surveys are another quantitative and qualitative tool used to track patient progress. The AOFAS and the Medical Outcomes Study SF-36 are most commonly used scales in patients with foot and ankle complaints.

The AOFAS rating system is made up of four scales for each specific region of the foot and ankle, such as hallux interphalangeal metatarsophalangeal, lesser metatarsophalangeal-interphalangeal, midfoot, and ankle-hindfoot.[71,72] Each regional scale includes self-reported data about pain and function. Although the AOFAS scale is more specific to the clinical area of concern unlike other scales, its reliability and validity has not been proven or endorsed.

Unlike AOFAS score, SF-36 is a more generic patient assessment tool used to cover a patient's overall health. SF-36 has lower levels of reliability and validity in regards to lower extremity assessment and lacks the sensitivity to capture clinical changes. Attempts to validate use of SF-36 in patients with lower extremity complaints failed by presenting results with lower sensitivities in musculoskeletal complaints than in regional systems.[71,72]

SooHoo and coworkers[72] called for a revised foot and ankle outcomes measures after showing poor association between the AOFAS and SF-36, especially in forefoot disorders than ankle-hindfoot conditions. The goal of revised scale should focus on the level of deformity, associated pain and stiffness, and overall impact on the patient's function. Capture of these data points could be used in conjunction with SF-36 to create a more thorough clinical picture of patients' foot ankle complaints.

To establish a reliable and validated self-assessment instrument that specifically measures patient symptoms and disability related to ankle OA, Domsic and Saltzman[73] devised an ankle OA scale (AOS) by modifying the Foot Function Index, a visual analog scale used to assess rheumatoid foot problems. Among 562 subjects diagnosed with unilateral ankle OA, the AOS showed excellent test-retest reliability with high degree of concordance with WOMAC and SF-36 scales. The AOS evaluated patients' subjective estimation of pain and disability related to ankle OA and was found to be a reliable and valid self-assessment instrument that specifically measures patient symptoms and disabilities related to ankle OA. AOS should play a role in monitoring the patient's progress postsurgical treatment of ankle OA.

Ankle fusion may be the gold standard for end-stage arthritis management in elderly patients; however, current interest in ankle joint replacements and implants can bring a more viable option for severe arthritis in younger patients without compromising the ankle joint motion. With the proliferation of new ankle implant designs, it is important to report accurate and reproducible data on the results of the various designs. That is the only way to adequately compare results.[69] Future outcome measurement studies are warranted to standardize and validate the use of ankle- and rearfoot-specific functional scales.

DISCUSSION

Ankle joint is a unique anatomic structure that encompasses anatomic and biomechanical features that distinguish it from the knee and hip joints. The talocrural joint is subjected to five times the body weight during stance,[30–34] yet the incidence of primary ankle OA is estimated in 1% of the population.[6,31] Talus has its functional paradoxes that make it an essential bony connection between the leg and the foot. This article introduces TTR, a surgical treatment option to highlight talus' distinct role within an ankle joint and introduces a discussion of 3D printed technology in the surgical arena.

Since initial introduction of TTR, there has been a resurgence of interest and modified applications of 3D printed anatomic structures. The most recent report demonstrated successful limb salvage through the use of a custom 3D printed titanium scaffold to replace significant tibial segmental bone loss with concomitant talus fracture.[74] Cartilage engineering found new hope in templates with complex interconnected bidirectional 3D printed microchannel networks to accelerate bone healing compared with untreated control subjects and showed comparable levels of bone healing versus bone matrix protein-2 administration.[75]

There are multiple applications for a total talar implant, because its use is reported in comminuted talar fracture and talar body tumor,[18] talar collapse after total ankle arthroplasty in a patient with rheumatoid arthritis,[12] talar AVN, talar OM, and ankle degenerative joint disease (DJD). The strength of these implants has an unpredictable lifespan but it has significant advantages over TAR and ankle fusion, especially in young and active patients.

How Does Talar Prosthesis Fare with Total Ankle Replacement?

On the heels of successful total hip and knee replacements, TAR instilled ambition into surgeon's hearts until the first series of disappointing outcomes was revealed. Early degeneration of the ankle systems, osteolysis, hardware loosening, and migration plagued TAR patients during 1980s. Total ankle arthroplasty enthusiasts lost their momentum and returned to a more predictable outcome achieved with ankle arthrodesis in 1990s. The early 2000s showed a near even split between TAR and arthrodesis procedures with the advent of newer TAR models.

Typical TAR failures stem from improper patient selection, implant style, or combination of the two. A patient's medical comorbidities, such as peripheral arterial disease and diabetes, along with history of smoking can jeopardize the outcome from the start. Improper surgical planning and execution affect TAR implant survival. For example, position of the STAR implant depends on proper talar component placement and thickness of the mobile bearing implant. Any inappropriate deviation in either component may lead to abnormal dorsiflexion and plantarflexion of the ankle joint.[76] Size mismatch, loosening, and subsidence of the TAR components contribute to a problem cycle of perpetuating further joint damage. The initial length of the deep fin in the STAR implant compromised talar precarious blood supply, which resulted in stem modification and improved patient outcomes.[38] In addition, postoperative complications, such as soft tissue infections, bone fractures, and poor compliance, can also contribute to TAR failure.

Most of the total ankle system designs failed because of talar component subsidence. Individual or combination of risk factors, from obesity, poor bone stock, to excessive bone resection during surgery,[15] contributed to the structural disintegration of the bone, and therefore lead to TAR component loosening. Despite the introduction of bone cement to improve component stability, most TAR models were ultimately destined for mechanical failure because of poor biomechanical understanding of the ankle joint.

The introduction of mobile bearing designs eliminated implant loosening and accelerated wear and stress on the bone implant interfaces. Consequently, major strides were undertaken to improve mechanical properties of the implants, which ultimately led to custom prosthesis.

One of the first attempts to create patient-specific talar body implant was documented in 1997 by Harnroongroj and Vanadurongwan[17] for treatment of talar AVN using contralateral ankle imaging. Eight out of nine patients evaluated at 15-year postoperative check-up reported satisfactory result. The ninth patient sustained talar stem loosening and migration into the talar neck that required revisional procedure.

With the advent of 3D printing, TTR made it more feasible to match the anatomy of the talus and its communications with the surrounding joints. Talus fits firmly between the navicular, calcaneus, tibia, and fibula. Close to 60% of the talus is covered with articular cartilage and it bears no muscular attachments.[24] Therefore, the talus is well-seated in the ankle joint and has little motion to protect itself from dislocation. Even without muscular attachments, talus depends on the congruous nature of the adjacent joints and integrity of the surrounding ligaments to support anatomic shape of the bone within an ankle joint.[17]

Based on this knowledge, total talus replacement success depends on congruence of adjacent articular surfaces and ligamentous stability of the ankle, subtalar, and talonavicular joints. Therefore to maintain close anatomic relationship, researchers have developed many ways to customize the implant, such as the addition of porous coating at the site of major ligaments (ie, deltoid),[24] augmenting the implant with use of Stryker internal brace in major ligamentous injuries based on preoperative MRI,[26] and reproducing anatomic congruence with the prospect of maintenance of the physiologic ankle joint ROM.[67]

Total talus implant was developed as a salvage procedure in young and active patients who did not meet the criteria for TAR and ankle fusion. Full recognition must be given to TTR as a promising treatment option for treatment of severe ankle joint arthritis, avascular necrosis, osteochondral lesions, and infectious bone disease, yet, it may not prolong the inevitable future ankle arthroplasty or arthrodesis.

Why Arthrodesis Is a Poor Procedure in a Young, Active Patient

Arthrodesis remains the gold standard for treatment of end-stage arthritis. The goal of any surgical fusion, whether it is ankle, tibiocalcaneal with bone block, or tibiotalocalcaneal arthrodesis, is to create pain-free plantigrade foot with solid union of the ankle. Multiple approaches have been described to achieve fusion, including internal and external fixation, each with its own risks and benefits. Although early attempts at ankle fusion were marked by high nonunion rates, especially those with large intercalary bone grafts, improvements in technique and materials have led to better outcomes.[21,31]

Contraindications to the procedure include significant peripheral arterial disease, poorly controlled diabetes, poor nutritional status, and tobacco abuse.[22] A retrospective study by Frey and colleagues[77] discovered a 41% ankle nonunion rate, with most patients undergoing fusion to address post-traumatic arthritis. Perlman and Thordarson[78] studied 67 ankle fusions performed to address post-traumatic arthritis and reported a 28% nonunion rate, with trend toward significance in those who smoked, abused alcohol, abused illicit drugs, had diabetes, and had psychiatric disorders. Zarutsky and colleagues conducted a study on the use of circular wire external fixation in the treatment of salvage ankle arthrodesis and reported a 51.2% major complication rate, with 17.7% of the patients developing unstable nonunion and 9.8% stable pseudoarthrosis after initial salvage surgery. In addition, Cobb and colleagues[79] reported that although the actual risk of nonunion after ankle fusion could not be established in their study, the relative risk was approximately four times greater for the patients who were smokers at surgery.

Management of the absent talar body in a posttraumatic setting has consisted of either a Blair type fusion when the talar head and neck are present, or tibiocalcaneal fusion when the entire talus is missing.[80] Arthrodesis of the tibia to the calcaneus has a lower union rate and has been reported at approximately 80%.[32,33] One group of authors used cancellous autograft to replace the absent talus in three cases with successful incorporation and good functional outcomes.[34] Even if successful union is achieved, the loss of limb length is certain and has been reported up to 4 cm.[43] The obligatory shortening of the limb leads to compensatory mechanisms that include pelvic tilt and increased knee flexion of the long extremity and equinus compensation on the short extremity.[37] Several authors have associated leg inequality with back pain, knee dysfunction, and OA of the hip,[6,47,53,54] thus suggesting near anatomic limb length restoration of the injured limb may help alleviate future degeneration of affected joints. The inconsistent union rate and/or altered mechanical relationships with either a Blair fusion or tibiocalcaneal fusion and the morbidity associated with large autograft harvest, led to consider alternative methods of reconstruction in the patient with an absent talar body.[50]

Although arthrodesis of the ankle achieves acceptable function, it eliminates the motion of the ankle and pseudarthrosis may develop. For this reason, tibiocalcaneal fixation supplemented with iliac crest bone graft is indicated in some cases of extensive osteonecrosis of the talar body.[23] Tibiocalcaneal arthrodesis with an allograft or autograft can address the problem of the limb length discrepancy by re-establishing functional limb length. The approach, however, has often been complicated by nonunion and graft collapse.[44] Furthermore, despite the benefit of a better take, the autograft has been associated with donor site morbidity in less than or equal to 48% of cases.[44] The noted complications have included, but are not limited to, chronic pain, fracture, hematoma, hypoesthesia, and wound dehiscence. Patients have reported more pain, in the short-term, at the donor site than at the surgical site. Other shortcomings have included the potential for graft collapse and a limited quantity of iliac crest autograft available.[1,44] Tibiotalocalcaneal arthrodesis with talectomy provides a functional plantigrade foot and effectively eliminates joint pain; however, it has the disadvantage of shortening the limb if the bone deficit is large.

Other options, such as TTR, benign neglect, or use of vascularized bone graft, are considered for talar pathologies. Among autografts and allografts and their disadvantages, 3D printing may replace reliance on the grafts. Reimplantation offers the following advantages relative to arthrodesis: retained joint space height and bone stock, which can contribute to improved hindfoot function and ankle joint mechanics. Replacement of the necrotic talus with an artificial total talus maintains leg length and joint function. Because the talus has complicated joint surfaces with surrounding bones, custommade implants are ideal for adjusting the joint, producing stability, preventing degenerative changes in adjacent joints, and dispersing the pressures appropriately.

REFERENCES

1. Cohen MM, Kazak M. Tibiocalcaneal arthrodesis with a porous tantalum spacer and locked intramedullary nail for post-traumatic global avascular necrosis of the talus. J Foot Ankle Surg 2015;54(6):1172–7.
2. Lee KB, Cho SG, Jung ST, et al. Total ankle arthroplasty following revascularization of avascular necrosis of the talar body: two case reports and literature review. Foot Ankle Int 2008;29(8):852–8.
3. Apostle KL, Umran T, Penner MJ. Reimplantation of a totally extruded talus: a case report. J Bone Joint Surg Am 2010;92(7):1661–5.
4. Smith CS, Nork SE, Sangeorzan BJ. The extruded talus: results of reimplantation. J Bone Joint Surg Am 2006;88(11):2418–24.
5. Koller H, Assuncao A, Kolb K, et al. Reconstructive surgery for complete talus extrusion using the sandwich block arthrodesis: a report of 2 cases. J Foot Ankle Surg 2007;46(6):493–8.
6. Chou LB. Orthopaedic knowledge update: foot and ankle 5. American Academy of Orthopedic Surgery; 2014. p. 107–28.
7. Gross CE, Haughom B, Chahal J, et al. Treatments for avascular necrosis of the talus: a systematic review. Foot Ankle Spec 2014;7(5):387–97.
8. Gross CE, Sershon RA, Frank JM, et al. Treatment of osteonecrosis of the talus. JBJS Rev 2016;4(7) [pii:01874474-201607000-00002].
9. Assal M, Stern R. Total extrusion of the talus. J Bone Joint Surg Am 2004;86: 2726–31.
10. Regauer M, Lange M, Soldan K, et al. Development of an internally braced prosthesis for total talus replacement. World J Orthop 2017;8(3):221–8.
11. Lee HS, Chung HW, Suh JS. Total talar extrusion without soft tissue attachments. Clin Orthop Surg 2014;6(2):236–41.
12. Tsukamoto S, Tanaka Y, Maegawa N, et al. Total talar replacement following collapse of the talar body as a complication of total ankle arthroplasty: a case report. J Bone Joint Surg Am 2010;92(11):2115–20.
13. Rzesacz EH, Culemann U, Illgner A, et al. Homologous talus replacement after talectomy in infection and septic talus necrosis. Experiences with 3 cases. Unfallchirurg 1997;100(6):497–501 [in German].
14. Lampert C. Ankle joint prosthesis for bone defects. Orthopade 2011;40(11): 978–83 [in German].
15. Conti SF, Wong YS. Complications of total ankle replacement. Foot Ankle Clin 2002;7(4):791–807.

16. Ketz J, Myerson M, Sanders R. The salvage of complex hindfoot problems with use of a custom talar total ankle prosthesis. J Bone Joint Surg Am 2012;94(13): 1194–200.

17. Harnroongroj T, Vanadurongwan V. The talar body prosthesis. J Bone Joint Surg Am 1997;79-A(9):1313–22.

18. Harnroongroj T, Harnroongroj T. The talar body prosthesis: results at ten to thirty-six years of follow-up. J Bone Joint Surg Am 2014;96:1211–8.

19. Magnan B, Facci E, Bartolozzi P. Traumatic loss of the talus treated with a talar body prosthesis and total ankle arthroplasty. A case report. J Bone Joint Surg Am 2004;86(8):1778–82.

20. Taniguchi A, Takakura Y, Sugimoto K, et al. The use of a ceramic talar body prosthesis in patients with aseptic necrosis of the talus. J Bone Joint Surg Br 2012; 94(11):1529–33.

21. Ando Y, Yasui T, Isawa K, et al. Total talar replacement for idiopathic necrosis of the talus: a case report. J Foot Ankle Surg 2016;55(6):1292–6.

22. Angthong C. Anatomic total talar prosthesis replacement surgery and ankle arthroplasty: an early case series in Thailand. Orthop Rev (Pavia) 2014;6:5486.

23. Taniguchi A, Takakura Y, Tanaka Y, et al. An alumina ceramic total talar prosthesis for osteonecrosis of the talus. J Bone Joint Surg Am 2015;97(16):1348–53.

24. Stevens BW, Dolan CM, Anderson JG, et al. Custom talar prosthesis after open talar extrusion in a pediatric patient. Foot Ankle Int 2007;28(8):933–8.

25. Tanaka Y, Takakura Y, Kadono K, et al. Alumina ceramic talar body prosthesis for idiopathic aseptic necrosis of the talus. Bioceramics 2002;15:805–8.

26. Giannini S, Cadossi M, Mazzotti A, et al. Custom-made total talonavicular replacement in a professional rock climber. J Foot Ankle Surg 2016;55(6):1271–5.

27. Belvedere C, Cadossi M, Mazzotti A, et al. Fluoroscopic and gait analyses for the functional performance of a custom-made total talonavicular replacement. J Foot Ankle Surg 2017;56(4):836–44.

28. Burston JL, Brankov B, Zellweger R. Reimplantation of a completely extruded talus 8 days following injury: a case report. J Foot Ankle Surg 2011;50(1):104–7.

29. Mulfinger GL, Trueta J. The blood supply of the talus. J Bone Joint Surg Br 1970; 52(1):160–7.

30. Daniels T, Thomas R. Etiology and biomechanics of ankle arthritis. Foot Ankle Clin 2003;85(5):923–36.

31. Valderrabano V, Horrisberger M, Russell I, et al. Etiology of ankle osteoarthritis. Clin Orthop Relat Res 2009;467(7):1800–6.

32. Burdett R. Forces predicted at the ankle during running. Med Sci Sports Exerc 1981;14:308–16.

33. Brockett CL, Chapman GJ. Biomechanics of the ankle. Orthop Trauma 2016; 30(3):232–8.

34. Saltzman CL, Salamon ML, Blanchard GM, et al. Epidemiology of ankle arthritis: report of consecutive series of 639 patients from a tertiary orthopaedic center. Iowa Orthop J 2005;25:44–6.

35. Huch K, Kuettner KE, Dieppe P. Osteoarthritis in ankle and knee joints. Semin Arthritis Rheum 1997;26(4):667–74.

36. van Dijk CN, Reilingh ML, Zengerink M, et al. Osteochondral defects in the ankle: why painful? Knee Surg Sports Traumatol Arthrosc 2010;18(5):570–80.

37. Segal AD, Shofer J, Hahn ME, et al. Functional limitations associated with end-stage ankle arthritis. J Bone Joint Surg Am 2012;94(9):777–83.

38. Oppermann J, Franzen J, Spies C, et al. The microvascular anatomy of the talus: a plastination study on the influence of total ankle replacement. Surg Radiol Anat 2014;36(5):487–94.
39. Tennant JN, Rungprai C, Pizzimenti MA, et al. Risks to the blood supply of the talus with four methods of total ankle arthroplasty: a cadaveric injection study. J Bone Joint Surg Am 2014;96(5):395–402.
40. Prasarn ML, Miller AN, Dyke JP, et al. Arterial anatomy of the talus: a cadaver and gadolinium-enhanced MRI study. Foot Ankle Int 2010;31(11):987–93.
41. Azar FM, Beaty JH, Canale ST. Campbell's operative orthopaedics. 13th edition. [Chapter: 88]. Philadelphia: Mosby; 2017. p. 4294–7.
42. Hawkins LG. Fractures of the neck of the talus. J Bone Joint Surg Am 1970;52: 991–1002.
43. Valmassy RL. Clinical biomechanics of the lower extremities. Elsevier; 1996. p. 2–8.
44. Demetriades L, Strauss E, Gallina J. Osteoarthritis of the ankle. Clin Orthop Relat Res 1998;349:28–42.
45. Curtis MJ, Michelson JD, Urquhart MW, et al. Tibiotalar contact and fibular malunion in ankle fractures. A cadaver study. Acta Orthop Scand 1992;63(3):326–9.
46. Thomas RH, Daniels TR. Ankle arthritis. J Bone Joint Surg Am 2003;85(5):923–36.
47. Takakura Y, Tanaka Y, Kumai T, et al. Low tibial osteotomy for osteoarthritis of the ankle. Results of a new operation in 18 patients. J Bone Joint Surg Am 1995; 77(1):50–4.
48. Takakura Y, Takaoka T, Tanaka Y, et al. Results of opening-wedge osteotomy for the treatment of a post-traumatic varus deformity of the ankle. J Bone Joint Surg Am 1998;80(2):213–8.
49. Macko VW, Matthews LS, Zwirkoski P, et al. The joint-contact area of the ankle: the contribution of the posterior malleolus. J Bone Joint Surg Am 1991;73:347–51.
50. Lindsjo U. Operative treatment of ankle fracture-dislocations. A follow-up study of 306/321 consecutive cases. Clin Orthop Relat Res 1976;199:28–38.
51. Harstall R, Lehmann O, Krause F, et al. Supramalleolar lateral closing wedge osteotomy for the treatment of varus ankle arthrosis. Foot Ankle Int 2007;28(5):542–8.
52. Marsh JL, Buckwalter J, Gelberman R, et al. Articular fractures: does an anatomic reduction really change the result? J Bone Joint Surg Am 2002;84(7):1259–71.
53. Garras DN, Raikin SM. Supramalleolar osteotomies as joint sparing management of ankle arthritis. Seminars in Arthroplasty 2010;21(4):230–49.
54. Ramsey PL, Hamilton W. Changes in tibiotalar area of contact caused by lateral talar shift. J Bone Joint Surg Am 1976;58(3):356–7.
55. Adelaar RS, Madrian JR. Avascular necrosis of the talus. Orthop Clin North Am 2004;35(3):383–95, xi.
56. Blair HC. Comminuted fractures and fracture dislocations of the body of the astragalus: operative treatment. Am J Surg 1943;59:37–43.
57. Dennison MG, Pool RD, Simonis RB, et al. Tibiocalcaneal fusion for avascular necrosis of the talus. J Bone Joint Surg Br 2001;83(2):199–203.
58. Dennis MD, Tullos HS. Blair tibiotalar arthrodesis for injuries to the talus. J Bone Joint Surg Am 1980;62(1):103–7.
59. Mann RA, Chou LB. Tibiocalcaneal arthrodesis. Foot Ankle Int 1995;16(7):401–5.
60. Dabov GD. Osteomyelitis. In: Canale ST, Beaty JH, editors. Campbell's operative orthopaedics. Philadelphia: Mosby; 2013. p. 764–87.
61. Joseph TN, Myerson MS. Use of talectomy in modern foot and ankle surgery. Foot Ankle Clin 2004;9(4):775–85.
62. Mohammad HR, Pillai A. Limb salvage talectomy for 3C Gustilo-Anderson fracture. J Surg Case Rep 2016;2016(5) [pii:rjw081].

63. Choi YR, Jeong JJ, Lee HS, et al. Completely extruded talus without soft tissue attachments. Clin Pract 2011;1(1):e12.
64. Detenbeck LC, Kelly PJ. Total dislocation of the talus. J Bone Joint Surg Am 1969; 51:283–8.
65. Canale ST, Kelly FB. Fractures of the neck of the talus. Long-term evaluation of seventy-one cases. J Bone Joint Surg Am 1978;60:143–56.
66. Brewster NT, Maffulli N. Reimplantation of the totally extruded talus. J Orthop Trauma 1997;11:42–5.
67. Leardini A, O'Connor JJ, Catani F, et al. Mobility of the human ankle and the design of total ankle replacement. Clin Orthop Relat Res 2004;(424):39–46.
68. Yoshinaga K. Replacement of femoral head using endoprosthesis (alumina ceramics vs metal)–an experimental study of canine articular cartilage. Nihon Seikeigeka Gakkai Zasshi 1987;61(5):521–30.
69. Coetzee JC, Castro MD. Accurate measurement of ankle range of motion after total ankle arthroplasty. Clin Orthop Relat Res 2004;(424):27–31.
70. Paley D, Herzenberg JE, Tetsworth K, et al. Deformity planning for frontal and sagittal plane corrective osteotomies. Orthop Clin North Am 1994;25:425–65.
71. Kitaoka HB, Alexander IJ, Adelaar RS, et al. Clinical rating systems for the ankle-hindfoot, midfoot, hallux, and lesser toes. Foot Ankle Int 1994;15:349–53.
72. SooHoo NF, Shuler M, Fleming LL. Evaluation of the validity of the AOFAS clinical rating systems by correlation to the SF-36. Foot Ankle Int 2003;24:50–5.
73. Domsic RT, Saltzman CL. Ankle osteoarthritis scale. Foot Ankle Int 1998;19(7): 466–71.
74. Hamid KS, Parekh SG, Adams SB. Salvage of severe foot and ankle trauma with a 3D printed scaffold. Foot Ankle Int 2016;37(4):433–9.
75. Daly AC, Pitacco P, Nulty J, et al. 3D printed microchannel networks to direct vascularisation during endochondral bone repair. Biomaterials 2018;162:34–46.
76. Tochigi Y, Rudert MJ, Brown TD, et al. The effect of accuracy of implantation on range of movement of the Scandinavian Total Ankle Replacement. J Bone Joint Surg Br 2005;87(5):736–40.
77. Frey C, Halikus NM, Vu-Rose T, et al. A review of ankle arthrodesis: predisposing factors to nonunion. Foot Ankle Int 1994;15(11):581–4.
78. Perlman MH, Thordarson DB. Ankle fusion in a high risk population: an assessment of nonunion risk factors. Foot Ankle Int 1999;20(8):491–6.
79. Cobb TK, Gabrielsen TA, Campbell DC 2nd, et al. Cigarette smoking and nonunion after ankle arthrodesis. Foot Ankle Int 1994;15(2):64–7.
80. Schuberth JM, Jennings MM. Reconstruction of the extruded talus with large allograft interfaces: a report of 3 cases. J Foot Ankle Surg 2008;47(5):476–82.

Treatment Strategies and Frame Configurations in the Management of Foot and Ankle Deformities

Alexander M. Cherkashin, MD[a],*, Mikhail L. Samchukov, MD[a],
Franz Birkholts, MD[b]

KEYWORDS

- Circular external fixation • Hexapod frame configurations • Foot and ankle
- Hexapod assemblies • Classification • Ring fixation • Deformity correction

KEY POINTS

- Despite the widespread use of hexapod circular external fixation for fracture reduction and bone deformity correction, there is no common nomenclature/classification of frame assemblies.
- We propose a unique approach to making the decision on whether to use a hexapod or Ilizarov-type fixator based on the correction, complexity, and ability to achieve the correction acutely.
- Various hexapod frame configurations for foot and ankle deformity correction were combined into a classification based on correction levels, fixation blocks, and direction of the strut attachments.
- This classification allows the combination of foot and ankle frame assemblies into a few standard hexapod configurations irrespective of which external fixator is used.
- Using the proposed nomenclature, this classification can be further expanded to include nonhexapod frames.

INTRODUCTION

G. Ilizarov laid the basis for a revolutionary way to treat foot and ankle deformities using various external fixation assemblies. His method has increased in popularity and evolved significantly over the last decades. The success of the method is based on

Disclosure Statement: No benefits in any form have been received from a commercial party related directly or indirectly to the subject of this article. All three of the authors are paid educational consultants for the medical device companies mentioned in the text.
[a] Texas Scottish Rite Hospital for Children, 2222 Welborn Street, Dallas, TX 75219, USA; [b] Walk A Mile Centre, 223 Clifton Avenue, Lyttelton, Pretoria 0157, South Africa
* Corresponding author.
E-mail address: Alex.Cherkashin@tsrh.org

Clin Podiatr Med Surg 35 (2018) 423–442
https://doi.org/10.1016/j.cpm.2018.05.003
0891-8422/18/© 2018 Elsevier Inc. All rights reserved.

podiatric.theclinics.com

an extremely flexible approach to the external stabilization of tibia and foot bones. The Ilizarov system is very versatile and allows for an almost infinite number of frame configurations, using a lot of components to permit an accurate solution of every foot pathology.[1,2] Unfortunately, this versatility has its negative side—for each particular foot pathology, the surgeon has to build these assemblies from scratch, often using a great number of different components.[1,3] Because of this limitation, newer advances in the circular external fixator technology, namely hexapod fixators, have developed.

These fixators provide the ability to accurately adjust the bone fragment position in all 3 axes by adjusting just the length of 6 interconnecting struts. The 6 struts that connect the rings are arranged in a specific configuration creating a parallel kinematic system or Stewart-Gough platform.[4,5] Parallel in this description means that correction of the position can be performed simultaneously (parallel) in all directions. Therefore, these fixators provide accurate simultaneous 3-dimensional adjustments of fragment position across a variety of clinical indications, including fracture management, deformity correction, limb lengthening, and joint arthrodesis. The ability to simultaneously correct complex deformities make hexapod frames especially attractive to manage foot and ankle deformities, where it is very rare that there is only 1 level of 1-plane deformity.[5–8] Severe deformities like recalcitrant clubfoot, neurologic foot, collapsed Charcot foot, and posttraumatic sequelae are examples of these complex foot and ankle problems that can be managed using hexapod external fixators.[8–10]

Despite the obvious advantages of the hexapod fixators, there are certain difficulties in building and adjusting these frames. Foot deformity correction is especially challenging, because these complex multiplanar deformities often require multiple levels of correction in quite a limited space. Despite the ease of hexapod strut adjustment, frame design and construction can be complex. Very often, because of severe deformity, the frame configuration is altered, and the fixator may be even too small to fit 6 struts.

All of these limitations result in difficulties in communication between surgeons and complicate the learning of these techniques. First attempts to standardize the nomenclature and description of the hexapod frames for foot and ankle were attempted by Taylor.[6,7] In an attempt to describe these quite elaborate constructs he brought some carpentry terms into the external fixation (miter or butt constructs) and even more colloquial frame names like Tennessee torpedo.[5,11]

Takata and colleagues[12] presented foot hexapod assemblies classification based on the frame position relative to the foot, orientation of the axis of the hexapod, and direction of the struts attachment to the reference ring. This classification seems quite ambiguous, because very similar assemblies were classified differently. Also, it is extremely difficult to use this classification with other hexapod systems.

Another level of difficulty is introduced with the necessity to use software to plan correction. The software requires the measurement and entry of 3 sets of parameters (deformity, mounting, and correction parameters). Using an algorithm, the software calculates when and how to adjust each of the 6 struts at each level of correction.[6,7] These instructions are then available to the patient as a prescription or adjustment schedule.

MODULAR CLASSIFICATION OF FOOT AND ANKLE DEFORMITY CORRECTION AND FRAMES ASSEMBLIES

The absence of common nomenclature brings the need to introduce a novel circular fixator design classification that encompasses all possible frame adaptations without the use of colloquial terms. There is also a need for a simple decision-making algorithm to decide when and why a hexapod frame can be more beneficial than a traditional Ilizarov-type fixator. Therefore, we propose a new modular approach to foot and ankle frame design. The basis of this approach is in dividing the bony structures of the foot and ankle into 4 dynamic blocks. These major anatomic blocks are (**Fig. 1**):

- Tibia,
- Talus,
- Calcaneus, and
- Forefoot.

This division is dynamic because the number of anatomic structures combined into each of the blocks varies depending on treatment goals. These anatomic blocks in turn can be combined in various fixation units, when 2 or 3 blocks are fixed together in 1 external fixation module. The second part of the approach is a simple decision-making algorithm of when to choose a hexapod frame over an Ilizarov-type circular fixator (**Fig. 2**).

After making a decision that existing foot and ankle pathology requires external fixation as a treatment modality, the following set of question helps to select which device might be more appropriate.

1. Is there a need for deformity correction?
    Very often the external fixator is used just as a simple stabilization frame:
    a. Spanning fixator to hold fracture fragments in place.
    b. Off-loading fixator to eliminate pressure on soft tissues after plantar ulcer repair.
    c. Joint-stabilization frame to aid in wound coverage after muscle flaps or bone grafts.
    For all of the above the answer is no, then a static Ilizarov Fixator is the solution.
2. If the answer is yes, a second question is: Can the deformity correction be done acutely?
    Acute correction is always preferable if soft tissue, blood vessels, and nerve tension can allow it. Examples include:
    a. Fracture reduction with external fixator.

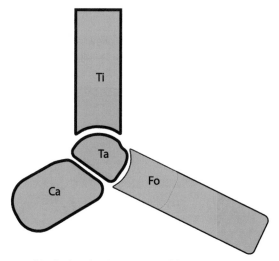

Fig. 1. Major anatomic blocks for the description of foot and ankle deformities. Ca, Calcaneus; Fo, forefoot (can be farther subdivided into midfoot and metatarsals); Ta, talus; Ti, tibia.

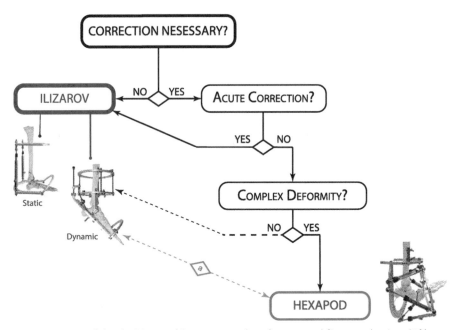

Fig. 2. Diagram of the decision-making process when for external fixator selection. [a] If hexapod struts don't fit - use hinges first and then fit in the struts.

    b. Resection of the nonunion and acute reduction.

    c. Osteotomy followed by an acute deformity correction of a malunion.

If the correction can be done acutely, it is also best to use the Ilizarov static fixator. However, very often initial acute correction can require some adjustments later on. To avoid problems later, it is suggested in those cases to use hexapod rings with rapid-adjust struts (TrueLok, Orthofix, Verona, Italy). In case additional gradual correction is needed later on, hexapod struts can be added to the frame and an additional gradual correction program can be run (**Fig. 3**). The TL-Hex hexapod system (Orthofix) allows for fast and simple exchange between Ilizarov-type connections into a hexapod reduction module.[13–16]

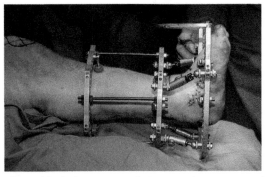

Fig. 3. Static frame for ankle fusion. Hexapod rings are interconnected by 4 rapid-adjust struts. These rapid adjust struts can be replaced by 6 hexapod struts for additional gradual deformity correction.

3. If the answer to the second question is no, then a third question is asked: Is there a complex deformity?

  If the answer is no, then an Ilizarov dynamic frame with hinges and an angular distractor is chosen. Again, for the same reason stated, we prefer to attach the hinges and distractor to the hexapod ring to provide for the ability to use more precise correction if necessary. Also, if a hexapod fixator is available, it is recommended to use it even for a "simple" 1-plane deformity correction (hence, a dotted line in the diagram).

When the answer is yes, then this is a clear indication to use hexapod-type external fixator.

- There is also one additional modifier to the selection for the hexapod fixator. If there is a need for gradual correction of complex deformity, but the segment (foot or tibia) is too small and/or deformity is too big to fit 6 struts in between the 2 rings, it is recommended to start with the hinges and correct the most significant part of deformity. This maneuver brings the hexapod rings into a more parallel position, which may allow to fit the struts and continue with more precise correction using a software program.

The third part of our approach is a standard description of the external fixator frame based on number of correction levels in between the anatomic blocks (discussed elsewhere in this article) and the orientation of the common vector of connecting struts.[17] Correction level is a separation between anatomic blocks (joint, osteotomy, nonunion site), which is bridged by the connection elements (struts). Struts are connected to the fixation blocks, which are attached to the corresponding anatomic blocks (**Fig. 4**).

- If the struts are bridging the correction level in a vertical direction the frame is labeled as 6V. Indications for the 6V frames are tibial deformity correction, ankle deformity correction, and so on.

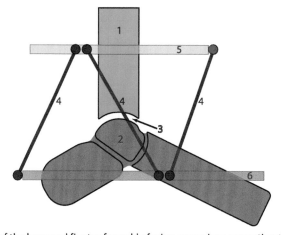

Fig. 4. Diagram of the hexapod fixator for ankle fusion or equinus correction through the ankle joint. 1, proximal anatomic block (tibia); 2, distal anatomic block (in this case it is entire foot); 3, correction level (ankle joint); 4, six hexapod struts bridging the correction level; 5, proximal fixation block (in this case it is 1 hexapod ring); 6, distal fixation block (in this case it is a hexapod foot plate). Reference segment and reference ring are shown in blue. Red dot represents ring orientation tab, always located on the reference ring between struts #1 and #2.

- If the general direction of struts bridging the correction level is horizontal (which is often happens in the foot frames), those frame are labeled as 6H. Midfoot Charcot deformity correction, calcaneal deformity correction through the osteotomy, and others are indications for the 6H frames.

When there is more than one correction level, the hexapod modules can be arranged in 3 different orientations:

1. Inline (double-level vertical or double-level horizontal);
2. Orthogonal (1 vertical hexapod module connected to a horizontal hexapod block); and
3. Parallel (2 parallel vertical frames).

When 2 hexapod blocks are stuck together, they may share the ring in between 2 correction levels, or each level can have its own set of 2 rings connected only to the struts spanning each level.

- In case of a shared ring, the ring in between the correction levels has 12 struts attached to it: 6 struts from one level and other 6 from the other level. If there are just 2 vertically oriented sets of struts this configuration is described as 6V × 6V, where the multiplication sign (×) illustrates the shared ring in between the stacks.
- If each level of correction has its own pair of rings connected with a set of struts and there is no common ring – these configurations have plus sign (+) illustrating that there is some static connection in between 2 middle rings of the stacked hexapod correction modules. Those 2 vertical frames without a shared ring would be described as 6V + 6V.
- In rare situations, there are 2 sets of struts are connected each to one of the 2 frames placed next to each other in a parallel manner. Those parallel frames and are descried as 6V ‖ 6V. In this configuration, 2 proximal rings from both hexapod modules are usually interconnected, and each set of struts moves corresponding distal ring independently.

The classification of the most common hexapod assemblies for foot and ankle are presented in **Fig. 5**.

SINGLE-LEVEL VERTICAL 6V FRAME

A single-level vertical 6V frame is the most often used hexapod assembly for the single-level deformity correction in upper or lower extremities. In foot and ankle applications, this construct is used for cases where the correction level located at the distal tibia or ankle joint (**Fig. 6**).

Indications

- Tibial and pilon fracture reduction.
- Tibial multiplanar deformity correction and/or lengthening (periarticular deformities, malunion, nonunion, leg length discrepancy, etc).
- Correction through ankle or subtalar joint with or without fusion.

Assembly

Basically, the frame consists of proximal and distal fixation blocks (each block can be a single hexapod ring or a hexapod ring attached to another support for increased stability) and 6 struts spanning the correction level. If deformity correction is performed through the ankle joint, the entire foot is fixed as a single anatomic block. A hexapod

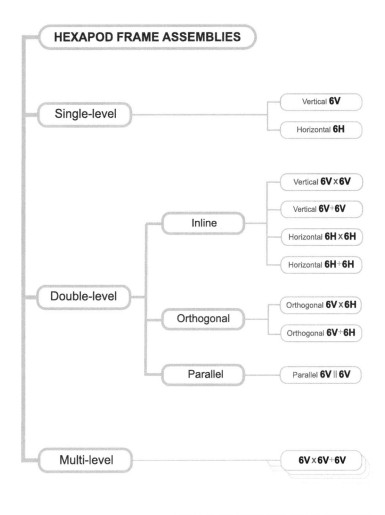

Fig. 5. Classification of the most common hexapod assemblies.

foot plate or a fixation block with foot plate and hexapod ring can be used to stabilize the foot (**Fig. 7**). In case when correction is performed through the subtalar joint, there is a need for additional stabilization of the talus as a single anatomic block with tibia (**Fig. 8**).

Software

TL-Hex software allows the ability to plan preoperatively and prebuild the frame before surgery. This feature is extremely helpful in cases with tibial deformity correction. However, when doing corrections through ankle or subtalar joints (equinus contractures, ankle distraction, et.) it is usually recommended to undertake the so-called rings first method, where the frame is applied first and then the deformity and mounting parameters are measured and entered into the software. The rings first method is used

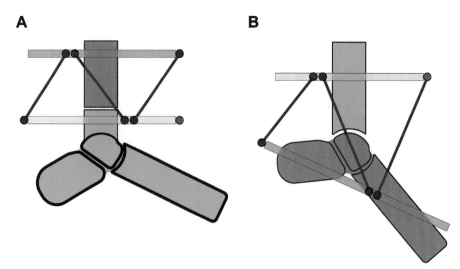

Fig. 6. Examples of the 6V frame configuration. (*A*) Distal tibial deformity correction. It is usually better to select distal reference segment (shown in *blue*) when performing distal tibial deformity correction. This step minimizes mistakes in measurement of mounting parameters. If the distal tibial segment is very short (periarticular deformity), it is usually recommended to include foot in frame, building 1 distal fixation block with hexapod ring attached to the distal tibia and foot plate attached to the foot. (*B*) Equinus correction through the ankle joint. The tibia is used as a reference segment. The entire foot is moved as a whole and is labeled as moving (*green*) segment.

when some partial intraoperative correction is performed and preoperative deformity parameters are not valid after surgery. When planning equinus deformity correction, it is recommended to use ankle graphics from the TL-Hex software (see **Fig. 7**B).

SINGLE-LEVEL HORIZONTAL 6H FRAME

The single-level horizontal 6H frame is most often used hexapod assembly for the single-level deformity correction of the foot (**Fig. 9**). In this assembly, the tibia and part of the foot (usually the talus, calcaneus, and midfoot) are fixed as one anatomic block. The rest of the foot (usually the forefoot) is fixed in a separate ring. This

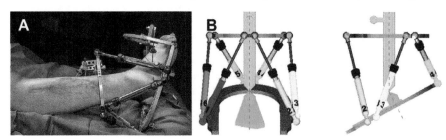

Fig. 7. The 6V hexapod frame used for ankle equinus deformity correction. (*A*) intraoperative picture of frame assembly. (*B*) TL-Hex software representation of the equinus deformity correction with the 6V hexapod. The tibia is usually used as a reference segment (shown in *blue*) and entire foot is used as one moving segment (shown in *green*). The tibia is selected as a reference because it is much easier to describe mounting of the proximal (reference) ring position relative to the axis of the tibia. The ring orientation tab is located on the reference ring (*red dot*).

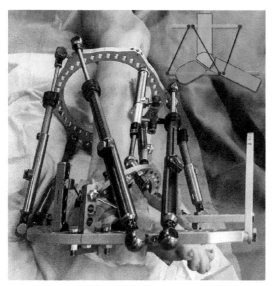

Fig. 8. Clinical example of the 6V hexapod frame used for the correction of the equinovarus deformity through subtalar and Chopart joints. Additional support is used to connect proximal (reference) ring to the talus, protecting the ankle joint and making talus a part of the proximal block along with the tibia. The diagram in the corner demonstrates anatomic blocks and level of correction. (*Courtesy of* J. Mostert, MB, Subiaco, Australia.)

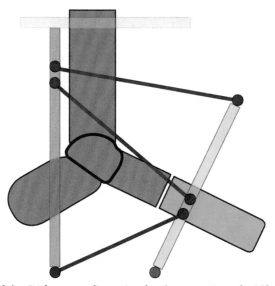

Fig. 9. Diagram of the 6H frame configuration for the correction of midfoot deformity. It is usually recommended to use distal reference because it is easier to enter mounting parameters in relation to the longitudinal axis of one of the metatarsal bones. Ring orientation tab (*red dot*) is located on the plantar side of the ring indicating 180° frame rotation. Part of midfoot, the talus, the calcaneus, and the tibia are stabilized as 1 block. This anatomic block is connected to 2 external supports mounted perpendicular (in a T-shaped configuration).

configuration is often referenced in the literature as a Butt frame,[5,6,11,18] derived from the carpentry term of perpendicular connection between 2 wooden blocks. Tibial ring and hindfoot support in this frame are often connected perpendicular to each other and work as a single unit.

Indications

- Lisfranc fracture-dislocation reduction.
- Midfoot deformity correction (Charcot midfoot protrusion, multiplanar midfoot/forefoot deformities), after acute correction of the hindfoot equinus, if present.
- Gradual calcaneal deformity correction, after acute correction of midfoot/forefoot deformity, if present.

Assembly

In the 6H configuration, both supports are connected more or less perpendicular to the longitudinal axis of the foot, resulting in a more horizontal alignment of the struts. Most often, the calcaneus is connected to a special open type support like a foot plate in the TL-Hex system or U-plate if using the TSF (Smith & Nephew, Memphis, TN). The open end of the support is attached in a perpendicular manner to the ring connected to the tibia (**Fig. 10**). The calcaneal foot plate is the proximal support and the forefoot ring is the distal support. The 6H frame can be thought of as a 6V frame laid on its back. The major difference is the absence of an anterior strut connection on the proximal support (there is an opening on the calcaneal support anteriorly). Because of the absence of the connection point for struts #1 and #2, it is usually recommended to attach these struts to the posterior tab of the proximal support. Because this point is used to reference frame orientation, this configuration will have a 180° rotation offset.

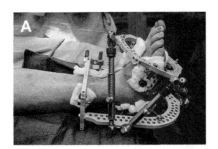

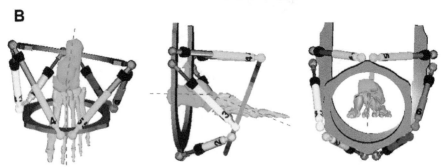

Fig. 10. The 6H frame for midfoot deformity correction. (*A*) Intraoperative picture. (*B*) TL-Hex software graphics showing distal reference segment (in blue color) and 180° of frame rotation. Distal reference ring mounting parameters are calculated relative to the axis of the second metatarsal. (*Courtesy of* L. Hlad, DPM, Columbus, OH.)

A similar frame configuration can be used for the gradual correction of hindfoot deformities owing to malposition of the calcaneus. After calcaneal osteotomy, a typical frame configuration in those cases comprises a T-shaped connection between the tibial ring and the anterior external support (foot plate) attached to the tibia/talus and posterior calcaneal external support (ring) interconnected by 6 struts.

Software

Some hexapod systems like the TL-Hex software allow the surgeon to choose special foot graphics to represent 6H frames for the foot deformity correction (see **Fig. 10B**). It is usually recommended to use distal referencing to plan the 6H assembly owing to ease of entering mounting parameters in relation to the longitudinal axis of one of the metatarsal bones. A major point to keep in mind is the 180° rotational frame offset. The TL-Hex software would automatically enter the 180° of external rotation of the frame as soon as the foot plate is confirmed as a selection for the proximal support.

DOUBLE-LEVEL HEXAPOD ASSEMBLIES

In the double-level frame configuration with 2 correction levels, 2 six-strut stacks are required. The most common configuration is an inline (series) configuration of the strut stacks, when both frames are either vertical (6V × 6V) or horizontal (6H × 6H) to each other. All double-level configurations require running 2 separate programs (one for each level of correction).

DOUBLE-LEVEL INLINE 6V × 6V AND 6V + 6V VERTICAL FRAMES

Double-level inline 6V × 6V and 6V + 6V vertical frames are the most frequent assemblies for double-level tibial deformity correction or for tibia and ankle joint deformity correction. These configurations are composed of 2 frames, stacked in series, lined up with the tibial axis, where each frame allows independent simultaneous repositioning of 2 bone segments relative to each other. The only difference between 2 vertical double-level frames is the presence or absence of the common ring (**Fig. 11**). If the distal ring on the proximal frame is also the proximal ring for the distal frame—this is the shared ring and frame is described as 6V × 6V. The shared ring has 12 struts attached to it—6 from each level. If the 2 frames do not share a common ring, this configuration is described as 6V + 6V.

Indications

- Double-level tibial deformity correction with or without lengthening.
- Bone transport in segmental tibial bone defects.
- Ankle fusion or tibiocalcaneal fusion simultaneously with tibial lengthening.
- Correction of complex foot and ankle deformities requiring realignment of the distal tibial segment relative to the proximal tibial segment simultaneously with hindfoot (whole foot) repositioning relative to the distal tibia (eg, equinus deformity of the foot due to combination of distal tibial procurvatum and ankle equinus contracture, etc).

Assembly

Two correction levels are separating either 3 tibial anatomic blocks or 2 tibial blocks and a foot. Typically, the double-level vertical frame consists of either 3 tibial fixation blocks (full rings or 5/8 rings) or 2 tibial and one whole foot fixation block (eg, foot plate) each interconnected by 2 sets of 6 struts.

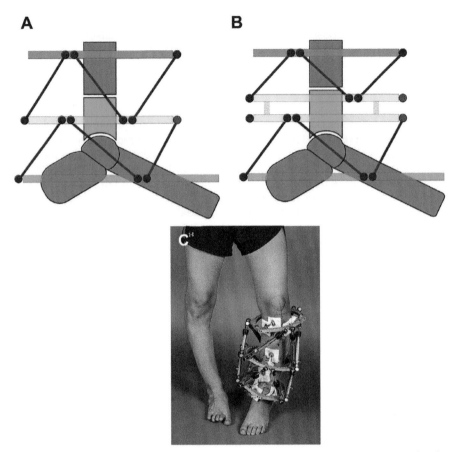

Fig. 11. Double-level vertical frames. (*A*) A 6V × 6V configuration. For the proximal level, a distal segment is used as a reference segment; however, if the tibial correction level is higher up in the tibia, the proximal referencing can be used. (*B*) A diagram of the 6V + 6V configuration. The middle segment on the tibia has double-ring block; therefore, there is no shared ring between 2 sets of hexapod correction modules. (*C*) Clinical photo of the 6V × 6V hexapod frame for double-level tibial deformity correction. The middle ring is shared between 2 levels of correction and has 12 struts attached to it (6 from each level).

Software

Two separate software programs run independently for each level of correction. It is like planning 2 independent 6V frames (see **Fig. 11**).

DOUBLE-LEVEL INLINE 6H × 6H AND 6H + 6H HORIZONTAL FRAMES

The double-level horizontally inline hexapod frame consists of 2 stacked frames, but they are lined up with the foot horizontal axis and allow independent simultaneous repositioning of 2 bone segments (forefoot and hindfoot) relative to the midfoot. The midfoot and tibia are combined in 1 anatomic block. These frames are quite bulky and often are larger than a patient's foot, requiring unconventional ways of being connected to the bone segments. Some of the hexapod systems with the dedicated strut attachment outside the external supports do not allow to share open-type supports like a foot plate. In such a situation, only a 6H + 6H frame configuration can be used (**Fig. 12**).

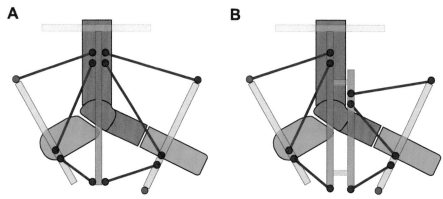

Fig. 12. Diagrams of the double-level horizontal frames. (*A*) The 6H × 6H configuration. For the proximal level of correction (calcaneal osteotomy) a proximal referencing is used, whereas for the distal level (midfoot osteotomy) the reference segment is distal. At the distal correction level, there is no dorsal tab on the proximal support; therefore, there is no place to connect struts #1 and #2. This factor is why the distal frame has rotation offset 180° similar to the single-level 6H frame for a midfoot deformity correction. (*B*) The 6H + 6H configuration, where there is no common middle ring between 2 frames. The fixation block consisting of one foot plate and one 5/8 ring open dorsally can be used to stabilize the middle anatomic block (tibia, talus and part of the midfoot).

Indications

- Two levels of foot deformity correction, where the talus or portion of the midfoot is connected to the tibia in one anatomic block and the hindfoot and forefoot are simultaneously repositioned relative to this middle block.
- Complex foot pathology (eg, equinocavovarus owing to a combination of hindfoot and forefoot deformities) requiring correction of the hindfoot position relative to the midfoot (tibia) simultaneously (or sequentially) with correction of the forefoot position relative to the midfoot (tibia).
- V- or Y-type osteotomies[1] for double-level complex foot deformity correction.

Assembly

This type of assembly can be visualized as two 6H frames connected together. Where one vertically oriented, open-type support is connecting midfoot and tibia forming a T-shaped construct and has 2 separate sets of struts one attached to forefoot and another one to the calcaneus. If the hardware used does not allow the simultaneous connection of 2 sets of struts to one foot plate or 5/8 ring (like TL-Hex foot plate), then 2 supports connected as a block should be used as an intermediate fixation module (**Fig. 13**A). Alternatively, nonconventional connections can be used (like emergency tabs in TL-Hex system).

Software

Two independent software programs are executed for the forefoot and hindfoot correction levels. In forefoot level, 180° frame rotation offset is used as in a 6H configuration. For the TL-Hex software, it is recommended to use foot dowels as a graphic representation of foot blocks. This step is recommended because the alignment of each anatomic foot block is done in relation to the midfoot, but not to each other (**Fig. 13**). Using a foot graphic in this situation would be rather more confusing than helpful.

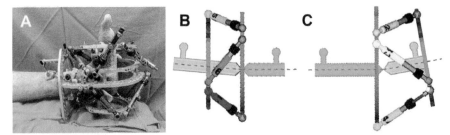

Fig. 13. The 6H + 6H frame configuration for double-level foot deformity correction through the V-osteotomy, using TL-Hex external fixator. (*A*) A middle anatomic block consisting of the tibia, the talus, the proximal portion of calcaneus, and the proximal part of the midfoot attached to the fixation block with a foot plate and a 5/8 ring. The foot plate is also connected to the other perpendicular foot plate holding tibial half-pins. (*B*) Software diagram for the forefoot correction with the distal part of the foot (*blue segment*) used as a reference segment with 180° frame rotation. (*C*) Software diagram for the calcaneal deformity correction, using the calcaneus as a proximal reference segment.

DOUBLE-LEVEL 6V × 6H AND 6V + 6H ORTHOGONAL FRAMES

The double-level orthogonal frame configuration represents 2 hexapods stacked at the angle to each other with the proximal frame lined up with the tibial axis and the distal frame lined up with the midfoot/forefoot horizontal axis. The most common 6V × 6H configuration has one common ring that is angulated relative to both the proximal (tibial) support and distal (foot) support (**Fig. 14**A). This configuration is often referenced in the literature as a miter frame, again derived from the carpentry term for the angular connection between 2 wooden blocks with an oblique joint.[5,6,11] In some

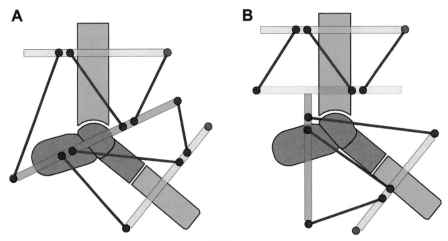

Fig. 14. Double-level orthogonal frames. (*A*) The 6V × 6V frame configuration. A proximal level of correction is at the ankle joint. A proximal segment (tibia) is used as a reference segment. A distal correction level is at the midfoot osteotomy. For the distal correction, distal referencing is used. (*B*) The 6V + 6V frame. Proximal correction level is also at the ankle joint, but the distal ring of the proximal module is not connected directly to the hindfoot. Instead, it connects to the perpendicular support to which calcaneus is attached. The distal ring of the proximal hexapod module has no attachment to the bones and acts as an intermediate support to control the position of the foot plate attached to it. Distal level of correction is similar to the standard 6H configuration.

situations, 2 perpendicular frames can be connected in a more complicated manner without an oblique shared ring in between 2 hexapod frames, described as 6V + 6H construct (**Fig. 14**B).

Indications

- Complex foot and ankle deformities requiring independent correction of the hindfoot position relative to the tibia simultaneously with correction of the forefoot position relative to the midfoot.
- Charcot midfoot collapse.
- Equinocavus deformity owing to a combination of hindfoot and forefoot malpositioning.

Assembly

The 6V × 6H configuration is one elegant and straightforward assembly (**Fig. 15**). It has a few limitations, however. First, it cannot be planned and preassembled preoperatively because the majority of the existing software does not allow for nonorthogonal placement of the nonreference ring. Second, if the proximal anatomic block includes both the ankle joint and the midfoot, additional stabilization for the talus is required inside the proximal frame (**Fig. 16**). In such a situation, it is probably better to try to work out placement of the 6H × 6H or 6H + 6H configuration. There is also some consideration in size and placement of the oblique shared ring; specifically, it is suggested to use a larger size ring than the ones for the tibial or forefoot supports. Also, when correcting the hindfoot equinus, sufficient ring inclination should be planned to avoid impingement on the tibia at the end of correction. Too much inclination can affect placement of the distal forefoot ring. Probably the safest way would be to use large enough ring and orient it parallel to the longitudinal axis of the calcaneus in lateral view (see **Fig. 15**).

The greatest advantage of the 6V + 6H over the miter frame is that it can be planned and preassembled preoperatively. In this configuration, the distal ring of the proximal hexapod module is actually not attached to any anatomic structures. It is a free-floating ring, which is connected to the proximal support of the distal horizontal frame. It is like taking the oblique shared ring of the 6V × 6H configuration and dividing it into 2 perpendicular rings while still controlling the same anatomic block of the hindfoot (see **Fig. 14**B).

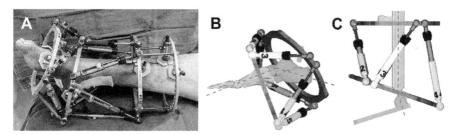

Fig. 15. The 6V × 6H hexapod frame. (*A*) The 6V × 6H frame configuration for the correction of ankle equinus and midfoot pronation-cavus deformity through the midfoot osteotomy. (*B*) Software diagram of the separate program for the distal level of correction. A distal segment (forefoot) is used as a reference. Foot graphic is used for better visualization of the planning. (*C*) Software diagram of the independent program for the proximal correction level. The tibia is used as a reference segment and an ankle diagram is selected to represent the hindfoot deformity.

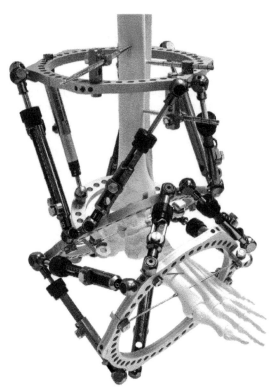

Fig. 16. The 6V × 6H frame for double level correction of the foot deformity, where the proximal anatomic block includes both ankle joint and midfoot. Additional stabilization of the talus is performed by placing half ring (with olive wire through the talus) inside the proximal hexapod module.

Software

For the 6V × 6H configuration, 2 independent programs are executed (see **Fig. 15**B–C). For the proximal frame, software is used the same way as for the 6V ankle frame. Ankle graphics with proximal referencing provides the best visualization when using the TL-Hex software. The distal portion is similar to running a 6H frame with 2 full rings construct and distal referencing. There is no need for the 180° rotation frame offset. As mentioned elsewhere in this article, this type of frame is usually applied as the ring first method.

In cases when preoperative planning and frame prebuilding is needed the 6V + 6H configuration is favored, it is suggested to run distal (foot) referencing for the proximal frame (**Fig. 17**). Distal referencing allows to place entire proximal frame above the ankle joint. The distal portion is planned similar to the 6H planning with distal reference ring and proximal open-type (5/8 ring) support.

DOUBLE-LEVEL 6V ‖ 6V PARALLEL FRAME

The double-level 6V ‖ 6V parallel frame is a less common frame configuration, where the 2 six-strut stacks are arranged parallel to each other in a vertical fashion. This is a quite bulky configuration that may be uncomfortable for patients (**Fig. 18**). However, it has the advantage of easy preoperative planning where deformities of hindfoot and forefoot are both referenced to the vertical axis of the tibia.

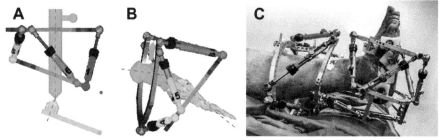

Fig. 17. Double-level correction of the ankle and foot deformity using orthogonal 6V + 6H frame configuration. (*A*) Software diagram of the proximal level of correction. If preoperative planning and frame preassembly is preferred, then distal referencing is necessary because it allows to position the reference ring above the ankle joint. (*B*) The separate software program for the midfoot deformity correction. At this level, distal referencing (forefoot) is used to plan the frame. (*C*) The 6V + 6H frame configuration for double-level deformity correction through the ankle joint and midfoot osteotomy. (*Courtesy of* T. O'Carrigan, FRACS, Norton, Australia.)

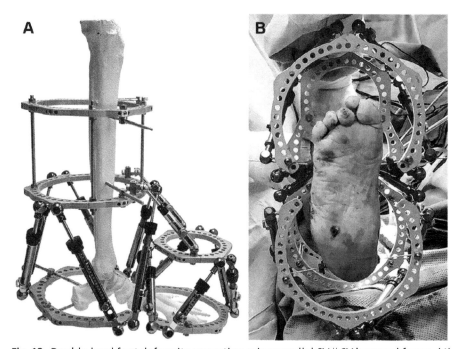

Fig. 18. Double-level foot deformity correction using parallel 6V || 6V hexapod frame. (*A*) Sawbones example of the 6V || 6V assembly. The tibial fixation block serves as a common fixation point for both hexapod modules. The distal ring of the hindfoot deformity correction module is connected with 6 vertical struts to the calcaneal fixation 5/8 ring. Second parallel 6V frame is connected to the same distal ring of the tibial block using rapid-adjust TrueLok struts. The proximal ring of this module does not have any direct connection to the tibia and distal ring is connected to the forefoot. (*B*) The 6V || 6V application for the rocker-bottom foot deformity correction. [*B*] *Courtesy of* Dr B. Wehrli, DPM, Rancho Mirage, CA.)

Indications

- Two levels of correction of hindfoot and forefoot deformities, where both deformities are referenced in relation to the vertical axis of the tibia.
- Equinocavovarus foot deformity, with equinus correction through the ankle joint and forefoot adduction and supination correction through midfoot osteotomy.
- Charcot complex foot deformity with 2 independent levels of correction: one through the ankle joint or calcaneal osteotomy and second through the midfoot osteotomy.

Assembly

Two parallel frames are attached to the tibia and the foot. The proximal ring from one (posterior) frame is attached to the tibia and interconnected by the 6 struts to the open support attached to the hindfoot. The proximal ring of the second (anterior) frame is connected to the proximal ring of the first frame and 6 struts from this ring are attached to the open support connected to the forefoot. In some hexapod systems, there is a special support (lobe support in TSF frame), which simplifies the interconnection between frames. When using the TL-Hex frame, the proximal ring from the anterior frame has to be mounted in such a way to allow for the strut attachment for both proximal supports (eg, to mount them on different levels).

Software

As for any double-level correction, 2 independent software programs run for each level of correction. The major difference in 6V ‖ 6V configuration is that both software programs use the tibia as a proximal reference. For the TL-Hex software, it is recommended to use the foot and ankle module of the software for better visual representation (**Fig. 19**).

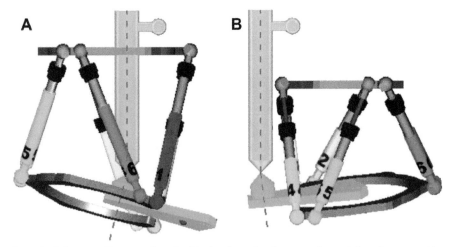

Fig. 19. Software diagram for double-level rocker-bottom foot deformity correction using 6V ‖ 6V hexapod frame configuration. Both software programs use tibia as proximal reference. (A) Hindfoot correction level. (B) Forefoot correction level. The tibia is used as a reference segment and frame is set to anterior offset, because the proximal (reference) ring is positioned anterior to the axis of the tibia.

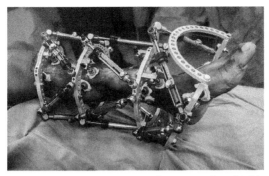

Fig. 20. A multilevel 6V × 6V × 6V hexapod configuration for tibial bone transport with simultaneous ankle equinus deformity correction.

MULTILEVEL FRAME CONFIGURATIONS

In the situations of multilevel deformities, especially in congenital deformities, more than 2 correction levels are often necessary to address the problem. Based on the previous examples, it should be obvious how to describe those configurations based on the orientation of common struts vector and connection between the hexapod modules (**Fig. 20**).

Very often, when dealing with complex multilevel deformities, hexapod correction blocks can be combined with Ilizarov-type hinges and simple lengthening rods. It is especially helpful in small pediatric extremities. In such situations, the presented classification can be extended to describe Ilizarov-type connections in between the fixation blocks. An example would be to depict the straight lengthening block as a 4V fixation (4 straight rods used for limb lengthening). A hinged system can be described as 3V (2 hinges and angular distractor for gradual deformity correction in vertical orientation). Extending this approach to include the description of any type of circular frame assembly would definitely help to standardize the nomenclature and simplify communication between surgeons.

SUMMARY

The Ilizarov fixator allows for almost unlimited configurations of external fixation frames to address different foot and ankle pathologies. Hexapod frames offer simplicity of adjustments and software helps to position a virtual hinge and proposes the necessary changes in length of 6 struts. However, this simplicity of frame assembly and adjustments does not limit the number of different frame configurations for the hexapod fixators. There remain many possible frame configurations, where similar deformities sometimes can be corrected using different hexapod frames.

The proposed standardized and rational approach to the external fixation frame assemblies and hexapod frame classification allows to facilitate decision-making guidelines to solve a variety of frame applications across different anatomic regions and different clinical scenarios. Described herein is a first attempt to standardize the indications and the structure of the frame that must be selected for each kind of deformity. We believe it can be developed further and help to define the clear description of any circular fixator for any particular problem.

REFERENCES

1. Kirienko A, Villa A, Calhoun JH. Ilizarov technique for complex foot and ankle deformities. New York: Marcel Dekker, Inc; 2004.

2. Paley D. The correction of complex foot deformities using Ilizarov's distraction osteotomies. Clin Orthop Relat Res 1993;293:97–111.
3. Ferreira RC, Costa MT. Recurrent clubfoot–approach and treatment with external fixation. Foot Ankle Clin 2009;14(3):435–45.
4. Akçali İD, Şahlar MO, Ün K, et al. A mathematical model in the implementation of a Stewart-Gough platform as an external fixator. In: Dössel O, Schlegel WC, editors. World congress on medical physics and biomedical engineering, September 7-12, 2009, Munich, Germany, 25/4. Berlin (Germany): Springer; 2009. IFMBE Proceedings.
5. Wukich DK, Belczyk RJ. An introduction to the Taylor spatial frame for foot and ankle applications. Oper Tech Orthop 2006;16(1):2–9.
6. Taylor J. TSF foot applications. 2002. Available at: http://www.jcharlestaylor.com/tsfliterature/08FootApps.pdf. Accessed February 28, 2018.
7. Taylor JC. Perioperative planning for two- and three-plane deformities. Foot Ankle Clin 2008;13(1):69–121, vi.
8. Young JL, Lamm BM, Herzenberg JE. Complex foot deformities: correction with the Taylor spatial frame. In: Kocaoğlu M, Tsuchiya H, Eralp L, editors. Advanced techniques in limb reconstruction surgery. Berlin (Germany): Springer; 2015. p. 377–405.
9. Waizy H, Windhagen H, Stukenborg-Colsman C, et al. Taylor spatial frame in severe foot deformities using double osteotomy: technical approach and primary results. Int Orthop 2011;35(10):1489–95.
10. Floerkemeier T, Stukenborg-Colsman C, Windhagen H, et al. Correction of severe foot deformities using the Taylor spatial frame. Foot Ankle Int 2011;32(2):176–82.
11. Dhar S. Ilizarov external fixation in the correction of severe pediatric foot and ankle deformities. Foot Ankle Clin 2010;15(2):265–85.
12. Takata M, Vilensky VA, Tsuchiya H, et al. Foot deformity correction with hexapod external fixator, the Ortho-SUV Frame™. J Foot Ankle Surg 2013;52(3):324–30.
13. Wilczek JL, LaPorta GA. The evolution of limb deformity: what has changed over the past ten years? Clin Podiatr Med Surg 2018;35(1):123–32.
14. Pesenti S, Iobst CA, Launay F. Evaluation of the external fixator TrueLok Hexapod System for tibial deformity correction in children. Orthop Traumatol Surg Res 2017;103(5):761–4.
15. Doudoulakis K. New kid on the block - the true look Hex frame: how does it compare to Taylor Spatial Frame? - Direct comparison of results in the treatment of severe open tibial fractures. Abstract # 174. Proceedings of ILLRS Congress Miami 2015 Combined Meeting of ILLRS, LLRS and ASAMI-BR. J Limb Lengthen Reconstr 2015;1(Suppl S1):1–117. Available at: http://www.jlimblengthrecon.org/article.asp?issn=2455-3719;year=2015;volume=1;issue=5;spage=1;epage=117;aulast=. Accessed March 5, 2018.
16. Ferreira N, Birkholtz F. Radiographic analysis of hexapod external fixators: fundamental differences between the Taylor Spatial Frame and TrueLok-Hex. J Med Eng Technol 2015;39(3):173–6.
17. Samchukov M, Cherkashin A, Birkholtz F. Classification of standard hexapod frame configurations, Abstract #42. Proceedings of ILLRS Congress Miami 2015 Combined Meeting of ILLRS, LLRS and ASAMI-BR. J Limb Lengthen Reconstr 2015; 1(Suppl S1):1–117. Available at: http://www.jlimblengthrecon.org/article.asp?issn=2455-3719;year=2015;volume=1;issue=5;spage=1;epage=117;aulast=. Accessed March 5, 2018.
18. Eidelman M, Katzman A. Treatment of arthrogrypotic foot deformities with the Taylor spatial frame. J Pediatr Orthop 2011;31(4):429–34.

Biomechanical Considerations in Foot and Ankle Circular External Fixation
Maintenance of Wire Tension

Check for updates

Mikhail L. Samchukov, MD[a],*, Craig E. Clifford, DPM, MHA[b],
Kevin M. McCann, DPM, MHA[c], Alexander M. Cherkashin, MD[a],
Byron Hutchinson, DPM[d], William A. Pierce, BS ENG[a]

KEYWORDS

- Circular external fixation • Foot and ankle • Foot frame biomechanics • Wire tension
- Calcaneal wire pretension • Metatarsal wire pretension • Wire tension loss

KEY POINTS

- Sequential tensioning of the calcaneal and metatarsal wires on foot support produces a reduction of transverse foot plate dimensions directly proportional to the magnitude of the wire tension.
- Regardless of the wire tensioning sequence or calcaneal cross-wire angle, anterior frame deformation is always considerably higher than the posterior frame deformation.
- Initial tension of primary wires is substantially preserved during forefoot wire pretension.
- Maximum preservation of the initial wire tension is achieved during the wire tension sequence with forefoot pretension, when the metatarsal wire is first tensioned to 130 kg, followed by sequential simultaneous tensioning of the calcaneal wires to 90 kg.
- Reduction in the initial wire tension can be decreased with utilization of more rigid double-row foot plates, especially when they are closed anteriorly via 2 transverse threaded rods.

Disclosure Statement: No benefits in any form have been received from a commercial party related directly or indirectly to the subject of this article. Three authors (M.L. Samchukov, B. Hutchinson, and A.M. Cherkashin) are paid educational consultants for the medical device company Orthofix mentioned in the text. In addition, B. Hutchinson is a paid consultant for medical device companies Integra and Paragon-28.
^a Texas Scottish Rite Hospital for Children, 2222 Welborn Street, Dallas, TX 75219, USA;
^b Franciscan Orthopedic Associates at St Francis, 34612 6th Avenue South, Suite 300, Federal Way, WA 98003, USA; ^c St Cloud Orthopedics, 1901 Connecticut Avenue South, Sartell, MN 56377, USA; ^d Franciscan Foot and Ankle Associates: Highline Clinic, 16233 Sylvester Road Southwest G-10, Seattle, WA 98166, USA
* Corresponding author.
E-mail address: mike@globalmednet.com

Clin Podiatr Med Surg 35 (2018) 443–455
https://doi.org/10.1016/j.cpm.2018.05.004
0891-8422/18/© 2018 Elsevier Inc. All rights reserved.

podiatric.theclinics.com

INTRODUCTION

Circular external fixation has become a prominent technique in the management of open diaphyseal and intra-articular fractures, malunions, nonunions, segmental bone and soft tissue defects, limb length discrepancies, joint contractures, and long bone deformities.[1–8] Circular fixators have several unique features not found in monolateral frames. Those characteristics include inherent multiplanar stability of bone segments and nonlinear axial stiffness provided by transosseous small-diameter tensioned wires alone or in combination with larger-diameter half pins.[9–16] Specifically, at low loads thin wires allow for a small amount of axial motion while becoming sufficiently stiffer to resist higher loads seen with weight bearing or under the distraction/compression forces. In addition, thin tensioned wires are much better tolerated by bone and soft tissues while providing stable but not too rigid fixation and promoting axial micromotion during weight bearing.[8,11–19]

With the recent popularization of the Ilizarov method and significant advances in osteotomy techniques, circular external fixation has gained increased utilization for severe foot and ankle deformity correction and complicated joint fusion. In those complex cases, this method provides superior adaptation of the fixation modules to abnormal anatomy of the foot while considerably improving segmental bone stabilization and long-term tolerance by soft tissues.[20–23]

External fixation of the foot is commonly accomplished by 2 calcaneal obliquely oriented cross wires and 1 or 2 transverse metatarsal wires, which are tensioned and secured to the external frame. Traditionally, the foot frame includes an open or closed U-shaped external support called a foot plate. Foot external support is then connected to the tibial ring or double-ring block via either 3 to 4 threaded or telescopic rods to create a static frame for acute foot repositioning or 6 hexapod struts to assemble a dynamic construct for gradual correction of foot and ankle deformities. Depending on the individual treatment objectives, soft tissue elasticity and alterations in bone anatomy and/or structure, stability of fixation can be further enhanced by insertion of additional wires through the metatarsals, midfoot, and/or talus.[1,4–6,20,21,24–27]

Design and assembly of appropriate external frame construct as well as spatial orientation of internal bone-stabilizing elements are an essential part of the treatment process for cases involving circular external fixation. Based on extensive experimental and clinical studies,[8,13,15,18,28–31] various extrinsic and intrinsic biomechanical parameters influence the stability of bone segment fixation within the external support. One of those important biomechanical parameters accountable for nonlinear stiffness of external fixation is the wire tension that should be maintained at the desired optimal level during the entire period of treatment.[2,8,13,14,17,19,32–35] In this regard, several factors are known to be responsible for the loss of initial wire tension, including wire yield due to repeated axial loading and wire slippage at the wire/fixation bolt interface.[16,33,36] Sequential tensioning of 2 wires attached to the same external support also caused significant alteration of their initial tension due to frame deformation.[17] To avoid the wire tension loss, some investigators suggested simultaneous tensioning of both wires attached to the same ring using 2 separate wire tensioners.[37]

Although numerous studies have addressed biomechanical characteristics of circular external fixation, they have mainly concentrated on the stabilization of the long bone. Biomechanical assessment of the parameters affecting the stability of circular external fixation in the foot and ankle is very limited[38] and does not include evaluation of the influence of wire tension sequence on the overall stability of the foot constructs and maintenance of achieved wire tension. Maintenance of the initial wire tension in the foot constructs, however, is critically important. Because 3 or more wires are most always used in the foot, their simultaneous tensioning is problematic. Moreover, some of those wires must be tensioned sequentially resulting in almost unavoidable foot plate deformation and reduction in the initial wire tension.

Therefore, the purpose of this study was to approach biomechanics of circular external fixation on the foot and evaluate multiple variables contributing to the loss of the initial hindfoot and forefoot wire tension within the most commonly used foot external supports. The authors' specific goal was to identify the effect of wire tension magnitude, calcaneal cross-wire angle and foot plate diameter, as well as foot plate rigidity, method of foot plate closure, and distance between the calcaneal and metatarsal wires on anterior and posterior foot plate deformation and the resulting reduction of the initial tension of the hindfoot/forefoot wires after sequential tensioning of opposing metatarsal/calcaneal wires.

BIOMECHANICAL TESTING

Mechanical testing was divided into 2 phases (**Table 1**). Phase I investigated the effect of wire tensioning sequence (calcaneal vs metatarsal wire pretension), tension magnitude of primary and secondary wires, calcaneal cross-wire angle, and transverse frame dimensions (foot plate diameter) on the anterior and posterior deformation of an external foot support and resulting loss of a primary wire initial tension. Phase II examined the influence of foot plate type, method of foot plate closure and distance between the metatarsal and calcaneal wires on frame deformation and wire tension loss using either metatarsal (phase IIA) or calcaneal (phase IIB) wire pretension.

In phase I (**Fig. 1**), a standard foot support consisting of an aluminum double-raw foot plate (TrueLok, Orthofix, Verona, Italy) closed anteriorly with a half ring were constructed in 150-mm-, 180-mm-, and 200-mm-diameter sizes. To simulate a typical clinical fixation pattern, 2 proximal hindfoot (calcaneal) cross wires intersecting each other at 56 mm distal to the posterior inside edge of the frame and one distal forefoot (metatarsal) transverse wire located 127 mm distal to the intersection of the calcaneal wires were attached to the constructed foot support using slotted wire fixation bolts.

Standard, smooth, 1.8-mm-diameter wires (TrueLok, Orthofix, Verona, Italy) were randomly chosen from the stock and modified for mechanical testing. A single linear strain gauge (Vishay Precision Group, Inc, Malvern, PA) was bonded to each wire in a uniform fashion using cyanoacrylate glue followed by an application of environmental epoxy coating (**Fig. 2**). The attached strain gauges were then instrumented to a strain gauge amplifier (Model 2120, Vishay Precision Group Inc, Malvern, PA) with the output connected to a digital multimeter. All strain gauge/wire units were individually calibrated by applying progressively increasing tensile loads within the previously established linear region from 20 kg to 175 kg using a servo-hydraulic mechanical testing system (Bionic 858, MTS Systems Corp, Eden Prairie, MN). For each strain gauge/wire unit, the calibration coefficient was obtained within the tensile load and the stress-strain curve was reviewed to ensure a linearity of the slope.

The wire tensioning sequence was alternated in 2 testing modes: forefoot (metatarsal) wire pretension and hindfoot (calcaneal) wire pretension. In the forefoot pretension sequence, the primary metatarsal wire was tensioned first, followed by simultaneous tensioning of the secondary calcaneal wires. In the hindfoot pretension sequence, the primary calcaneal wires were tensioned first followed by tensioning of the secondary metatarsal wire. In both sequences, the primary wires were tensioned to 90 kg, 110 kg, and 130 kg using a standard calibrated wire tensioner, whereas at each primary wire tension magnitude, the secondary wires were tensioned also to

Table 1
Phases of biomechanical testing and parameters tested

Testing Phase	Fixation Module	Parameters Tested
Phase I	There are 2 calcaneal wires crossing at variable angles and intersecting 56 mm distal to the posterior inside edge of the frame and one transverse metatarsal wire located 127 mm distal to the intersection of calcaneal wires. Wires are tensioned using a variable pretension sequence to variable tension magnitude and attached to variable diameter double-row foot plate closed anteriorly with half ring.	Wire pretension: calcaneal, metatarsal Primary wire tension (kg): 90, 110, 130 Secondary wire tension (kg): 90, 110, 130 Calcaneal cross-wire angle (°): 30, 45, 60 Foot plate diameter (mm): 150, 180, 200
Phase IIA	There are 2 calcaneal wires crossing at a 30° angle 56 mm distal to the posterior inside edge of the frame and one transverse metatarsal wire located at the variable distance from the calcaneal wires. Primary metatarsal wire is tensioned to 130 kg of initial tension followed by simultaneous tensioning of calcaneal wire to 90 kg. Wires are attached to 180-mm-diameter foot plate closed anteriorly with variable closure methods.	Foot plate: modular single row, rigid double row Closure: half ring, foot plate, threaded rods Distance b/w wires (mm): 97, 127, 157
Phase IIB	There are 2 calcaneal wires crossing at a 30° angle 56 mm distal to the posterior inside edge of the frame and one transverse metatarsal wire located 127 mm distal to the intersection of calcaneal wires. Primary calcaneal wires are simultaneously tensioned to 130 kg of initial tension followed by tensioning of the metatarsal wire to variable tension magnitude. Wires are attached to 180-mm-diameter foot plate closed anteriorly with variable closure methods.	Foot plate: modular single row, rigid double row Foot plate closure: half ring, threaded rods Metatarsal wire tension (kg): 90, 110, 130

90 kg, 110 kg, and 130 kg. Changes in the primary wire initial tension were monitored through attached strain gauges. In addition, the foot plate width was measured at its anterior and posterior sections (see **Fig. 1**B) before and after each trial of secondary wire tensioning; the difference was recorded as the anterior and posterior frame deformation. Testing of each experimental pair was repeated 3 times at 3 different (30°, 45°, and 60°) calcaneal cross-wire angles and 3 different (150 mm, 180 mm, and 200 mm) foot plate diameters.

Statistical analysis was performed using a paired 2-sample t-test (significance of $P<.05$) to compare percent changes in frame deformation and wire tension between the two tensioning sequences. A one-way analysis of variance (ANOVA) with Tukey post hoc tests (significance of $P<.05$) was used to compare changes in frame deformation and wire tension between foot support sizes, calcaneal wire-cross angles, and tension magnitudes.

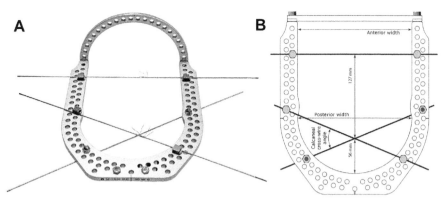

Fig. 1. Frame assembly for phase I biomechanical testing. (*A*) Standard frame construct consisting of double-row rigid foot plate closed anteriorly with half ring. (*B*) Location and orientation of metatarsal and calcaneal wires within the foot plate.

In phase II, 6 different frame configurations were tested (**Fig. 3**). Three of those frame assemblies consisted of a standard 180-mm-diameter single-row modular foot plate with plate extensions (see **Fig. 3**A), whereas the other 3 foot supports (see **Fig. 3**B) included a rigid double-raw foot plate (TrueLok, Orthofix, Verona, Italy). In each group, foot supports were closed anteriorly using a standard half ring, another single-row modular foot plate, or 2 threaded rods attached to the foot plate with the posts.

In all frame assemblies, 2 calcaneal wires were crossing at a 30° angle 56 mm distal to the posterior inside edge of the frame. A single transverse metatarsal wire was positioned across the anterior portion of each construct at distances of 97 mm, 127 mm, and 157 mm from the calcaneal wires. Initially (phase IIA), the forefoot pretension

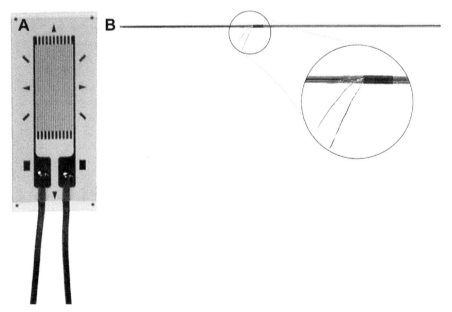

Fig. 2. Smooth 1.8-mm-diameter wire modified for biomechanical testing. (*A*) Close-up view of foil-alloy strain gauge. (*B*) The strain gauge bonded to the wire and epoxy coated.

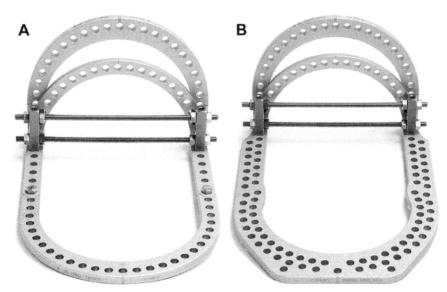

Fig. 3. Frame assemblies for phase II biomechanical testing. (*A*) Single-row modular foot plate with 2 plate extensions closed anteriorly with half ring, foot plate, or 2 threaded rods. (*B*) Double-row rigid foot plate closed anteriorly with half ring, foot plate, or 2 threaded rods.

sequence was applied to all assemblies with the primary metatarsal wire tensioned to 130 kg followed by simultaneous tensioning of the calcaneal wires to 90 kg. Similar to phase I, tension of the metatarsal wire was measured before and after tensioning of the calcaneal wires in order to calculate a percent change in primary wire tension. In addition, dimensions of each construct were measured at the anterior and posterior widths both before and after wire tensioning to assess construct deformation. Statistical analysis was performed comparing group means using one-way ANOVA with Tukey post hoc tests (significance of $P<.05$) to assess tension change as a result of foot plate type, metatarsal wire position, and closure method.

For further assessment (phase IIB), 3 selected constructs were tested with a reverse (calcaneal) pretension sequence including (1) a rigid double-row foot plate with half-ring closure, (2) a rigid double-row foot plate with threaded-rod closure, and (3) a modular single-row foot support with plate extensions and half-ring closure. In those assemblies, 2 primary calcaneal wires crossing at a 30° angle were simultaneously tensioned to 130 kg followed by tension of the secondary single metatarsal wire to 90 kg, 110 kg, and 130 kg.

MAINTENANCE OF INITIAL WIRE TENSION

The influence of various biomechanical parameters, including wire tension sequence and magnitude, calcaneal cross-wire angle, foot plate diameter, rigidity, and closure method, as well as the distance between the calcaneal and metatarsal wires on foot plate deformation and reduction of wire tension are presented on **Figs. 4–7**.

Wire Tensioning Sequence

Across all measurements, both metatarsal and calcaneal wire pretension resulted in frame deformation. Importantly, the tensioning sequence did not have a significant

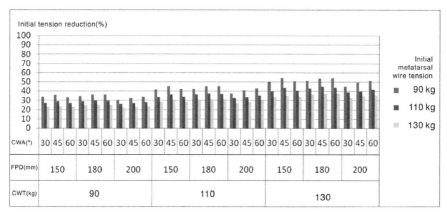

Fig. 4. Metatarsal wire initial tension reduction in forefoot pretension sequence. CWA, calcaneal wire angle; CWT, calcaneal wire sequential tension; FPD, foot plate diameter.

effect on overall changes in the anterior and posterior foot plate widths after wire tension. The average reduction in the posterior foot support dimensions during forefoot pretension was similar to that during calcaneal pretension averaging 0.76% ±0.13% and 0.75% ±0.12%, respectively ($P = .62$). Similarly, the deformation of foot support anteriorly was 2.13% ±0.36% when the forefoot wire was tensioned first and 2.4% ±0.32% during calcaneal wire pretension ($P = .13$).

Comparison of primary wire tension before and after secondary wire tensioning also indicated that sequential tensioning of the secondary wires produced a reduction in the initial tension of the opposing primary wires in both wire tensioning sequences. However, the initial tension of primary wires was greater preserved during forefoot wire pretension resulting in an average reduction of metatarsal wire tension on 35.9% ±8.18%. In the hindfoot pretension sequence, reduction of the initial tension of primary calcaneal wires following the sequential tensioning of the forefoot metatarsal wire was significantly ($P<.05$) higher averaging 61.0% ±12.3%.

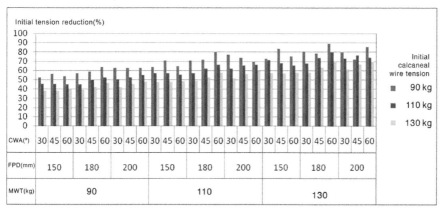

Fig. 5. Calcaneal wires initial tension reduction in hindfoot pretension sequence. CWA, calcaneal wire angle; FPD, foot plate diameter; MWT, metatarsal wire sequential tension.

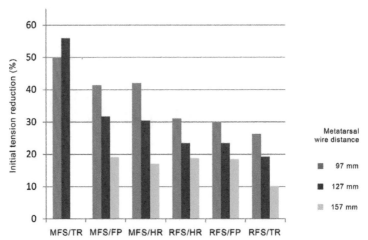

Fig. 6. Comparative reduction of metatarsal wire tension in single-row modular and double-row rigid foot supports closed anteriorly with half-ring, single-row foot plate or 2 threaded rods. MFS/FP, modular foot support with single-row foot plate; MFS/HR, modular foot support with half-ring; MFS/TR, modular foot support with threaded rods; RFS/FP, rigid double-row foot support with single-row foot plate; RFS/HR, rigid double-row foot support with half-ring; RFS/TR, rigid double-row foot support with threaded rods.

Wire Tension Magnitude

Regardless of tensioning sequence, wire tension magnitude showed significant influence ($P<.05$) on both anterior and posterior frame deformations. The average reduction in the anterior foot plate width, however, was significantly higher ($P<.05$) than that in the posterior width (range from 1.99%–2.55% and from 0.68%–0.84%, respectively) and directly proportional to the amount of wire tension.

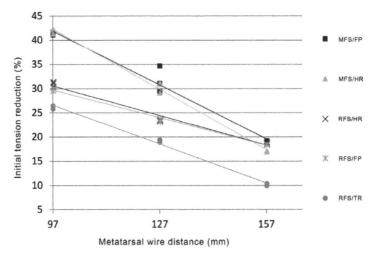

Fig. 7. Influence of distance between the metatarsal and calcaneal wires on metatarsal wire tension reduction. MFS/FP, modular foot support with single-row foot plate; MFS/HR, modular foot support with half ring; RFS/FP, rigid double-row foot support with single-row foot plate; RFS/HR, rigid double-row foot support with half ring; RFS/TR, rigid double-row foot support with threaded rods.

Analysis of wire tension magnitude demonstrated its significant effect on the maintenance of achieved wire tension. The maximum overall preservation of initial wire tension was observed during forefoot pretension sequence when the forefoot wire was tensioned first to 130 kg followed by sequential simultaneous tensioning of the calcaneal wires to 90 kg. This pairing in wire tension magnitude resulted in an average of 23.9% ±1.15% reduction of the initial forefoot wire tension and was significantly different from all other wire tension magnitude pairings ($P<.05$). The highest reduction of the forefoot initial wire tension during the forefoot pretension sequence was 51.3% ±2.85%, which occurred with an initial forefoot wire tension to 90 kg followed by tensioning of the calcaneal wires to 130 kg. Similarly, the initial tension of calcaneal wires to 90 kg followed by tensioning of the forefoot wire to 130 kg in the calcaneal pretension sequence resulted in the highest loss of the calcaneal initial wire tension (average 79.9% ±5.71%). The lowest initial wire tension loss in the calcaneal pretension sequence was 42.2% ±4.75% and observed in calcaneal wires tensioned to 130 kg followed by forefoot wire tension to 90 kg.

Foot Plate Diameter

Posterior transverse frame deformation was reversely proportional to the foot plate diameter showing a statistically significant difference ($P<.05$) between all 3 sizes of foot supports. Similarly, changes in anterior foot support width after wire tensioning revealed a significant difference ($P<.05$) between the 150-mm-diameter foot plate and both larger sizes indicating that the smaller frame is inclined to less anterior frame deformation. There was no significant difference, however, between the 180-mm- and 200-mm-diameter foot supports ($P = .19$), suggesting a size-dependent plateau effect in anterior frame deformation.

Interestingly, comparison of the initial wire tension loss between different sizes of foot supports showed no statistically significant difference in either forefoot or calcaneal wire pretension sequence. In forefoot pretension sequence, the average amount of the observed metatarsal wire initial tension loss was 35.7% ±8.52%, 37.7% ±8.28%, and 34.4% ±7.75% for 150-mm-, 180-mm-, and 200-mm-diameter foot plates, respectively ($P = .94$). Likewise, loss of calcaneal initial wire tension in the hindfoot pretension sequence was 56.9% ±11.89%, 62.4% ±13.14%, and 63.9% ±11.14% for the same sizes of foot plate, respectively ($P = .59$).

Calcaneal Cross-Wire Angle

Review of the initial wire tension loss in different calcaneal cross-wire angles demonstrated no statistically significant difference in both wire pretension sequences. In the forefoot pretension sequence, for example, the average amount of metatarsal wire initial tension loss was 34.7% ±7.79%, 36.67% ±8.6%, and 36.4% ±8.37% for 30°, 45°, and 60° calcaneal cross-wire angles, respectively ($P = .88$). The amount of the initial calcaneal wire tension loss in hindfoot pretension was 59.0% ±12.38%, 61.1% ±11.96%, and 63.1% ±12.68% for the same calcaneal cross-wire angles, respectively ($P = .99$). Similarly, there was no significant difference in either anterior ($P = .91$) or posterior ($P = .62$) frame deformation between the examined calcaneal cross-wire angles.

Foot Plate Rigidity

Biomechanical testing of different types of frame constructs revealed transverse deformation in all 6 assemblies. Foot supports with a more rigid double-row foot plate, however, produced significantly less ($P<.05$) anterior and posterior frame deformation compared with that in foot supports with a modular single-row foot plate. More likely, this difference occurred because of their flexibility at the bolts connecting them to plate extensions. The average anterior and posterior deformation of double-row foot plates, for example, was 0.05 mm ±0.05 mm and 0.25 mm ±0.09 mm, respectively, whereas the average anterior and posterior deformation of single-row modular foot plates was 0.72 mm ±0.51 mm and 1.23 mm ±0.38 mm, respectively.

Similarly, reduction of the initial metatarsal wire tension was observed in all tested constructs. Across all measurements, foot supports with a double-row foot plate showed significantly less (*P*<.05) loss in the initial wire tension than that in foot supports with a modular single-row foot plate (average 22.37% ±5.79% and 30.01 ±8.47%, respectively). Interestingly, the amount of the initial tension loss of the metatarsal wire was not correlated with either anterior or posterior frame deformation.

Additional testing of 3 constructs with a reverse (calcaneal) pretension sequence further reinforced those findings. Foot supports with more rigid double-row foot plate and threaded rod closure resisted calcaneal wire tension loss significantly better (12.31% ±2.24%) than the other constructs. The rigid double-row foot plate with a half-ring closure produced a mean wire tension loss of 48.78% ±8.25%, which was not significantly different from that (52.82% ±9.33%) in the modular foot support with a half-ring closure.

Finally, because the calcaneal wires were attached to the different surfaces of foot support (one wire on the same surface of the foot plate as the metatarsal wire and the other wire on the opposite surface of the foot support), they showed a different amount of the individual tension reduction after sequential tensioning of the metatarsal wire. This effect may result in a torsional bending of calcaneus within the foot support after tensioning of the metatarsal wire. In this regard, again the more rigid double-row foot plate with threaded rod closure demonstrated the minimal difference (2.66 kg) between the tension loss in both calcaneal wires, resulting in potentially the least torsional bending of the calcaneus. This difference in calcaneal wire tension loss was significantly different from that in the other constructs tested in the calcaneal wire pretension sequence.

Foot Plate Closure

Comparison of different foot plate closure methods for maintenance of the initial metatarsal wire tension demonstrated that the double-row foot plate with a threaded rod closure (**Fig. 8**) produced the highest resistance to wire tension loss (average 18.6%). The wire tension loss produced by the double-row foot plate with a threaded rod closure was significantly less (*P*<.05) than the wire tension loss observed in the foot supports consisting of a similar double-row foot plate with either a half-ring

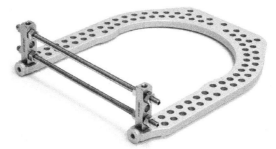

Fig. 8. Double-row rigid foot plate closed anteriorly with 2 threaded rods providing maximum preservation of metatarsal wire initial tension.

closure (average 24.49%) or single-row foot plate closure (average 24.06%). There was no significant difference found in wire tension preservation between those last two constructs.

Although the threaded-rod closure produced the maximum resistance to wire tension loss in the rigid double-row foot plate constructs, it resulted in the significantly highest metatarsal wire tension loss (an average 53.06%) in the modular foot plate assemblies with plate extensions.

Metatarsal-Calcaneal Wire Distance

Analysis of the influence of the distance between the metatarsal and calcaneal wires on the initial metatarsal wire tension strongly revealed the inverse linear relationship with a higher decrease in the initial tension in the metatarsal wires located more close to the calcaneal wires. Across all examined constructs, the mean wire tension reduction was on average 8.7% for each 30-mm decrease in the metatarsal-calcaneal wire distance. The exception to this tendency was the modular foot plate supports with threaded rod closure that did not show a statistically significant difference among different metatarsal wire positions.

CLINICAL IMPLICATIONS

Circular external fixation of the foot is commonly achieved by 2 calcaneal cross wires and one metatarsal wire sequentially tensioned and secured to the external foot plate. Two wire tension sequences are clinically applicable in foot stabilization: sequence with hindfoot pretention (initial simultaneous tensioning of calcaneal wires followed by tensioning of the metatarsal wire) and sequence with forefoot pretension (initial tensioning of the metatarsal wire followed by simultaneous tensioning of calcaneal wires).

Both wire tension sequences produce equal reduction in transverse foot plate dimensions directly proportional to the magnitude of wire tension. Regardless of wire tensioning sequence or calcaneal cross-wire angle, anterior frame deformation is always considerably higher than the posterior frame deformation, although both deformations are inversely proportional to foot plate diameter indicating that the smaller frame is inclined to less deformations.

Although both wire tension sequences caused similar foot frame deformation and resulted in a reduction in wire tension, the initial tension of primary wires is substantially greater preserved during forefoot wire pretension. Importantly, neither the calcaneal cross-wire angle nor foot plate diameter has noteworthy influence on the initial wire tension loss in both wire tension sequences.

Maximum preservation of the initial wire tension is achieved during the wire tension sequence with forefoot pretension when the metatarsal wire is tensioned first to 130 kg followed by sequential simultaneous tensioning of the calcaneal wires to 90 kg. Interestingly, the maximum loss of the initial wire tension in the presented biomechanical testing was detected in the reverse wire tension sequence to similar magnitudes with hindfoot pretension when the calcaneal wires were tensioned first to 90 kg followed by tensioning of the metatarsal wire to 130 kg.

Reduction in the initial wire tension can be further decreased with utilization of more rigid double-row foot plates (compared with single-row modular foot plates), especially when those plates are closed anteriorly via 2 transverse threaded rods attached to both ends of the foot plate by connecting posts. Foot plate closure using two transverse threaded rods allows manipulation with the amount of frame deformation and resulted final magnitude of wire tension. The amount of frame deformation can also be reduced by increasing the distance between the metatarsal and calcaneal wires.

REFERENCES

1. Brunner R, Hefti F, Tgetgel JD. Arthrogrypotic joint contracture at the knee and the foot. J Pediatr Orthop B 1997;6:192–7.
2. Calhoun JH, Li F, Ledbetter BR, et al. Biomechanics of the Ilizarov fixator for fracture fixation. Clin Orthop Relat Res 1992;280:15–22.
3. Cattaneo R, Catagni M, Johnson EE. The treatment of infected nonunions and segmental defects of the tibia by the methods of Ilizarov. Clin Orthop Relat Res 1992;280:143–52.
4. Dennison MG, Pool RD, Simonis RB, et al. Tibiocalcaneal fusion for avascular necrosis of the talus. J Bone Joint Surg Br 2001;83:199–203.
5. Grant AD, Atar D, Lehman WB. The Ilizarov technique in correction of complex foot deformities. Clin Orthop Relat Res 1992;280:94–103.
6. Hosny GA. Correction of foot deformities by the Ilizarov method without corrective osteotomies or soft tissue release. J Pediatr Orthop B 2002;11:121–8.
7. Paley D. The correction of complex foot deformities using Ilizarov's distraction osteotomies. Clin Orthop Relat Res 1993;293:97–111.
8. Wolfson N, Galpin RD, Hearn TC, et al. Control of interfragmentary micromotion in Ilizarov distraction osteogenesis. Bull Hosp Jt Dis 1992;52:36–8.
9. Nele U, Maffulli N, Pintore E. Biomechanics of radiotransparent circular external fixators. Clin Orthop Relat Res 1994;308:68–72.
10. Tucker HL, Kendra JC, Kinnebrew TE. Management of unstable open and closed tibial fractures using the Ilizarov method. Clin Orthop Relat Res 1992;280:125–35.
11. Ilizarov GA. The tension-stress effect on the genesis and growth of tissues: part II. The influence of the rate and frequency of distraction. Clin Orthop Relat Res 1989;239:263–85.
12. Goodship AE, Watkins PE, Rigby HS, et al. The role of fixator frame stiffness in the control of fracture healing. An experimental study. J Biomech 1993;26:1027–35.
13. Fleming B, Paley D, Kristiansen T, et al. A biomechanical analysis of the Ilizarov external fixator. Clin Orthop Relat Res 1989;241:95–105.
14. Kummer FJ. Biomechanics of the Ilizarov external fixator. Clin Orthop Relat Res 1992;280:11–4.
15. Bronson DG, Samchukov ML, Birch JG, et al. Stability of external circular fixation: a multi-variable biomechanical analysis. Clin Biomech 1998;13:441–8.
16. Aronson J, Harp JH. Mechanical considerations in using tensioned wires in a transosseous external fixation system. Clin Orthop Relat Res 1992;280:23–9.
17. Lewis DD, Bronson DG, Samchukov ML, et al. Biomechanics of circular external skeletal fixation. Vet Surg 1998;27:454–64.
18. Bronson DG, Samchukov ML, Birch JG. Stabilization of a short juxta-articular bone segment with a circular external fixator. J Pediatr Orthop B 2002;11:143–9.
19. Wu JJ, Shyr H, Chao E, et al. Comparison of osteotomy healing under external fixation devices with different stiffness characteristics. J Bone Joint Surg Am 1984;66:1258–64.
20. Ilizarov GA. Operative correction of foot deformities. In: Ilizarov GA, editor. Transosseous osteosynthesis. Berlin: Springer-Verlag; 1992. p. 583–634.
21. Koczewski P, Shadi M, Napiontek M. Foot lengthening using the Ilizarov device: the transverse tarsal joint resection versus osteotomy. J Pediatr Orthop B 2002;11:68–72.
22. Laughlin RT, Calhoun JH. Ring fixators for reconstruction of traumatic disorders of the foot and ankle. Orthop Clin North Am 2002;26:287–94.

23. Paley D. Principles of deformity correction. Berlin: Heidelberg: Springer-Verlag; 2002. p. 593–625.
24. Bradish CF, Noor S. The Ilizarov method in the treatment of relapsed clubfeet. J Bone Joint Surg Br 2000;82:387–91.
25. Catagni MA. Foot. In: Bianchi Maiocchi A, editor. Atlas for the insertion of transosseous wires and half-pins. Milan (Italy): Medi Surgical Video; 2002. p. 45–6.
26. Choi IH, Yang MS, Chung CY, et al. The treatment of recurrent arthrogrypotic club foot in children by the Ilizarov method. A preliminary report. J Bone Joint Surg Br 2001;83:731–7.
27. Johnson EE, Weltmer J, Lian GJ, et al. Ilizarov ankle arthrodesis. Clin Orthop Relat Res 1992;280:160–9.
28. Calhoun JH, Li F, Bauford WL, et al. Rigidity of half-pins for the Ilizarov external fixator. Bull Hosp Jt Dis 1992;52:21–6.
29. Kummer FJ. Biomechanics of the Ilizarov external fixator. Bull Hosp Jt Dis 1989; 49:140–7.
30. Podolsky A, Chao EYS. Mechanical performance of Ilizarov circular external fixators in comparison with other external fixators. Clin Orthop Relat Res 1993; 293:61–70.
31. Pugh KJ, Wolinsky PR, Dawson JM, et al. The biomechanics of hybrid external fixation. J Orthop Trauma 1999;13:20–6.
32. Aronson J, Harrison B, Boyd CM, et al. Mechanical induction of osteogenesis: the importance of pin rigidity. J Pediatr Orthop 1988;8:396–401.
33. Stein H, Perren SM, Mosheiff R, et al. Decline in transfixing K-wire tension of the circular external fixator: experimental continuous in vivo measurements. Orthopedics 2001;24:985–9.
34. Wolfson N, Hearn TC, Thomason JJ, et al. Force and stiffness changes during Ilizarov leg lengthening. Clin Orthop Relat Res 1990;250:58–60.
35. Antoci V, Voor MJ, Antoci V Jr, et al. Effect of wire tension on stiffness of tensioned fine wires in external fixation: a mechanical study. Am J Orthop 2007;36:473–6.
36. Aquarius R, Van Kampen A, Verdonschot N. Rapid pre-tension loss in the Ilizarov external fixator: an in vitro study. Acta Orthop 2007;78:654–60.
37. Antoci V, Voor MJ, Antoci V Jr, et al. Biomechanics of olive wire positioning and tensioning characteristics. J Pediatr Orthop 2005;25:798–803.
38. Rocchio TM, Younes MB, Bronson DG, et al. Mechanical effect of posterior wire or half-pin configuration on stabilization utilizing a model of circular external fixation of the foot. Foot Ankle Int 2004;25:136–43.

Essentials of Deformity Planning

Paul A. Stasko, DPM[a],*, Lee M. Hlad, DPM[b,c,1]

KEYWORDS

- Deformity • Deformity planning • Radiographic angles • Varus • Valgus
- Radiographic measurements • Osteotomy rules

KEY POINTS

- Physical examination of the entire lower extremity in dynamic and static phases is essential for a complete evaluation of a foot and ankle deformity.
- Radiographic evaluations should include pelvis, hips, knees, and ankles to provide practitioner with weightbearing analysis of joint and muscle influences.
- Deformity analysis should involve comprehensive knowledge of biomechanics as well as compensatory mechanisms of joints.

INTRODUCTION/HISTORY

Deformity planning is a process that is innate to even the most novice of surgeons. As we evaluate each patient clinically, we see a problem and can classify this as a deformity. It is how we come to this conclusion that needs to be reproducible and accurate. We each have different methods as to how we attain the end goal of deformity correction, and it is not the purpose of this article to change one's practice; however, it is the purpose to perhaps enhance the ability to achieve this quicker and with more reproducible outcomes. The authors discuss key elements to clinical evaluation, radiographic assessment, and osteotomy to better create that normal limb alignment.

CLINICAL EVALUATION

Physical examination of the entire lower extremity is essential for a complete evaluation of a foot and ankle deformity. There are instances whereby a foot and ankle deformity comes from compensatory mechanisms from a more proximal site; therefore,

Disclosure Statement: None.
[a] Podiatry-Foot and Ankle Surgery, Rochester Regional Health-Fingerlakes Bone and Joint Center, 875 Pre Emption Road, Geneva, NY 14456, USA; [b] Grant Medical Center, 11 S Grant Avenue, Columbus, OH 43215, USA; [c] Nationwide Children's Hospital, 555 South 18th Street, Columbus, OH 43205, USA
[1] Present address: 6670 Perimeter Drive, Dublin, OH 43016.
* Corresponding author.
E-mail address: Paul.A.Stasko@gmail.com

evaluation of the pelvis, femur, and tibia should be included with the ankle and foot. Practitioners should evaluate statically sitting, laying, and standing. Dynamic evaluation should be performed to see the soft tissue influences on the bone structure.

Goniometers may be thought of today as primitive tools but are a favorite to most planning surgeons. These simple devices are a lost art in today's ever changing digital world. Newer applications and programs allow for assistance in deformity planning but cannot replace basic knowledge when clinically assessing patients, and we must not forget about paper-doll cutouts and pen-and-paper drawings. Many planning modules for external fixators have software that is designed to use basic deformity parameters in assessing and finding the deformities. Inexpensive applications, such as Bone Ninja, can be a tool that allows a surgeon to, in real time, take pictures of radiographs or clinical deformities and perform the surgery in front of patients to see what the correction would be like. These programs can streamline deformity planning and allow images to be shared and discussed with colleagues. Whether you are using a digital device or pencil and paper, similar outcomes should be achieved and should ultimately allow the practitioner to isolate the deformity and pick the type of correction needed.

RADIOGRAPHIC ASSESSMENT

Radiographic assessment for most foot and ankle practices involved the ankle and below. Norms have been established regarding foot and ankle measurements.[1–12] It is essential in preparing for large deformity correction that proximal films be obtained to ensure no other influences are present. Commonly, long leg films should be obtained and evaluated. These radiographs are only possible if institutions have programs that allow stitching of the radiographs together or if they have full-length cassettes for radiographs that span from the pelvis to the floor. Practitioners should make sure they use a measuring device, whether it is a grid they place on the plate itself or a mag ball to allow for calibration. They should standardize their format with patella forward for all the films as well as accommodating with 1-cm heel lifts to make the pelvis even. Radiology technologists should be in tune with deformity and should understand the signs to watch for gross limb length discrepancy, including pelvic tilt, shoulder droop, and head tilt.

When assessing for a foot and ankle deformity, standard anterior posterior and lateral radiographs should be viewed. Additional films can be obtained with a calcaneal axial which and show frontal plan involvement but perhaps is better suited through Saltzman views, if clinics practices and equipment allow.[1,13] These views have been shown to allow the best visualization of the calcaneal tibial relationship.[9,14]

RADIOGRAPHIC EVALUATION

As stated before, radiographic assessment of deformity is crucial when planning procedures to correct the foot and ankle deformity. There are different planes that must be evaluated to objectively evaluate the magnitude of the deformity. For the sake of this article, pertinent radiographic angles are reviewed for the foot and ankle.

Ankle

Frontal plane analysis of the ankle is best suited with anteroposterior (AP) as well as mortise views. Care should be taken to include most if not all of the tibia in the film. The mortise view is often just to see congruity of the joint and is not normally used for angle measurements. The sagittal plane should be taken with medial malleoli against the cassette with the ankle at 90° (**Figs. 1** and **2**).

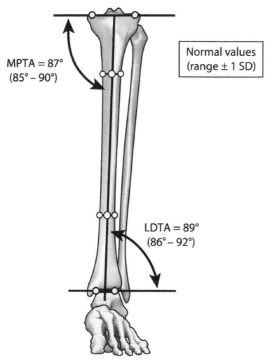

Fig. 1. Frontal plane analysis. LDTA, lateral distal tibial angle; MPTA, medial proximal tibial angle; SD, standard deviation. (*Courtesy of* Rubin Institute for Advanced Orthopedics, Sinai Hospital of Baltimore, Baltimore, MD, 2018; with permission.)

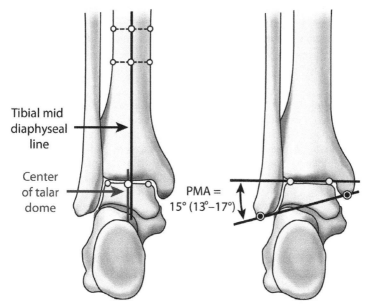

Fig. 2. Frontal plane analysis alternate. PMA, plafond malleolar angle. (*Courtesy of* Rubin Institute for Advanced Orthopedics, Sinai Hospital of Baltimore, Baltimore, MD, 2018; with permission.)

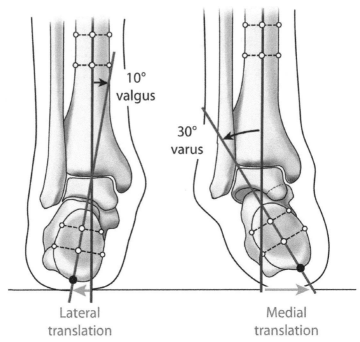

10°
valgus

30°
varus

Lateral
translation

Medial
translation

Fig. 3. Hindfoot alignment view. (*Courtesy of* Rubin Institute for Advanced Orthopedics, Sinai Hospital of Baltimore, Baltimore, MD, 2018; with permission.)

Foot/Hindfoot Alignment

Hindfoot alignment views, including Saltzman or calcaneal axial radiographs, are useful in hindfoot deformity correction and planning.[13] Tibiocalcaneal angle, foot height, and joint congruency are evaluated on these views. Anatomic axis of the tibial and calcaneus is used.[15] Hindfoot varus and valgus deformities are appreciated on these views. These views are critical in flatfoot and cavus surgery (**Figs. 3** and **4**).

TRANSVERSE PLANE
Foot

AP views of the foot are important in the evaluation a variety of foot deformities. From basic to advanced procedures, radiographic evaluation of the foot is essential to appreciate the correction that the surgeon needs. There are many important angles in this series using the anatomic axis of the foot bones. AP Meary angle (talo-first metatarsal) and talocalcaneal angle is essential in flatfoot deformity correction and analysis.[15] The first intermetatarsal and hallux abductus angle are critical in bunion surgery. Metatarsal parabola as well as joint congruency is evaluated on AP radiographic views[9] (**Fig. 5**).

SAGITTAL PLANE
Ankle

Lateral views of the ankle using the anatomic axis allow for procurvatum and recurvatum deformity evaluation. Evaluation of cases such as tibial malunion and equinus deformity can be measured. The anterior distal tibial angle is measured, and the anatomic axis that bisects the tibia can be used to find the apex of the deformity.[14,15] Joint congruency is measured, which is important in posttraumatic cases whereby the ankle joint has been involved.

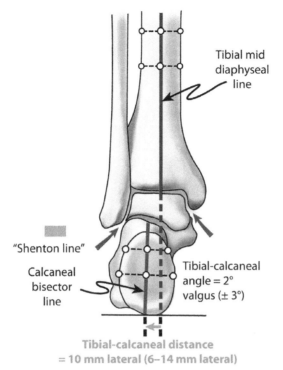

Tibial mid diaphyseal line

"Shenton line"

Calcaneal bisector line

Tibial-calcaneal angle = 2° valgus (± 3°)

Tibial-calcaneal distance = 10 mm lateral (6–14 mm lateral)

Fig. 4. Hindfoot alignment view alternate. (*Courtesy of* Rubin Institute for Advanced Ortho-pedics, Sinai Hospital of Baltimore, Baltimore, MD, 2018; with permission.)

Foot

Deformity planning in the sagittal plane in the foot is used for multiple foot deformities. Both flatfoot and cavus foot deformities will show abnormal calcaneal inclination angle, lateral Meary angle (talo-first metatarsal), and talar declination angle. Bisection of the talus and first metatarsal using the anatomic axis will show the apex of the defor-mity and can be used both preoperatively, postoperatively, and intraoperatively to appreciate correction of the deformity.[9,14,15] In cases involving midfoot osteotomy, the apex of the deformity can be used to determine the level of the osteotomy.

COMPENSATORY MECHANISMS

When deformity planning, knowledge of compensation mechanisms for the different planes is important for determining the underlying condition and choosing the surgical procedure. This section discusses compensation as it pertains to the foot.

Frontal Plane

Compensation of the frontal plane in the hindfoot is compensated by motion in the subtalar joint. When the full motion of the subtalar joint is used, compensation will then occur through the ankle joint. This compensation will lead to stress in various point of the ankle, which can lead to varus or valgus tilt of the ankle. Compensation can be seen in other parts of the foot as well. Hindfoot valgus can lead to compensa-tory forefoot supinatus. Hindfoot varus will create compensatory forefoot pronation, leading to a plantarflexed first metatarsal.

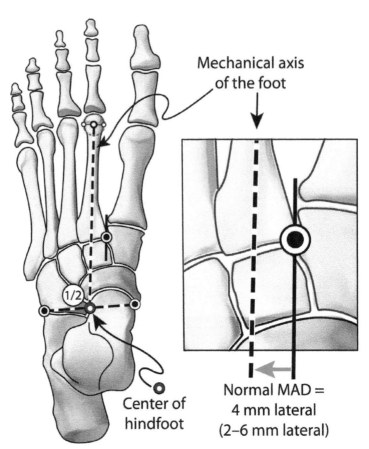

Mechanical axis of the foot

Center of hindfoot

Normal MAD = 4 mm lateral (2–6 mm lateral)

Fig. 5. AP views of the foot are important in the evaluation a variety of foot deformities. (*Courtesy of* Rubin Institute for Advanced Orthopedics, Sinai Hospital of Baltimore, Baltimore, MD, 2018; with permission.)

Sagittal Plane

In cases of procurvatum or recurvatum, deformity at the ankle will cause compensation in the foot and soft tissue of the lower leg. Recurvatum deformity of the ankle will cause distal displacement of the center of the ankle joint. The gastrocnemius-soleus complex can compensate for this by contracting, which can lead to equinus deformity and decreased plantarflexion strength of the Achilles tendon. In cases of flatfoot deformity, the forefoot will supinate in response to a decrease in calcaneal inclination angle. When dealing with cavus foot, hindfoot, forefoot, or combined cavus will determine which part of the foot is compensating.

Transverse Plane

Compensation for transverse plane deformities of the foot will occur at the level of the metatarsophalangeal joints (MPJs). Abduction or adduction of the metatarsals will cause deformity in the opposing direction at the level of the MPJs, which is seen in basic bunion deformity as well as metatarsus adductus.

Once radiographs have been taken, the practitioner must decide planal dominance and picking apex or center of rotation of angulation of deformity. Often deformities are in more than one plane and can be termed oblique plane deformities. After an apex is established the practitioner must determine how they are going to perform an osteotomy and by which method. Ultimately they are trying to reestablish a known alignment that places forces through the mechanical axis deviation (MAD) both through the ankle and the foot. In the foot this is defined as a point 4 mm lateral to the base of the second

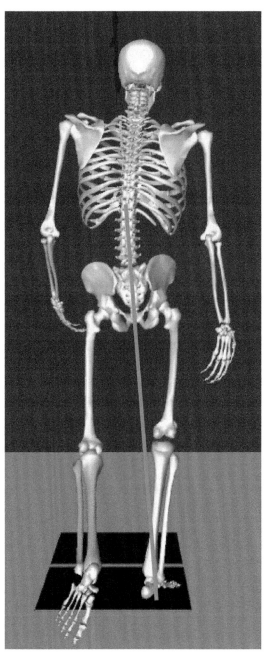

Fig. 6. They are trying to reestablish a known alignment that places forces through the MAD both through the ankle and the foot (*green line*). (*Courtesy of* Rubin Institute for Advanced Orthopedics, Sinai Hospital of Baltimore, Baltimore, MD, 2018; with permission.)

met articulation with the medial cuneiform and a line drawn from the center of the second metatarsal head to a central bisector line from a point half way between the calcaneal cuboid joint and the medial point of the talar navicular joint. The ground reaction vector of the ankle passes just lateral to the calcaneus from T10 (**Fig. 6**).

OSTEOTOMY

Osteotomy method and type is perhaps one of the most important concepts a practitioner must understand after finding the deformity. Rules of osteotomies are crucial to the success of the type of osteotomy and are paramount to practitioner understanding if they are going to do deformity correction. One must understand that in deformity planning sagittal plane assessment has to use anatomic evaluation only where in the frontal plane one can use mechanical or anatomic planning methods. Three general rules are involved with osteotomy. Rule 1 involves the osteotomy and axis of correction of angulation (ACA) are at the apex of the deformity the bone ends will align with angulation without any translation.[15,16] An example of this would be a closing wedge-type osteotomy. Osteotomy rule 2 is that when the correction of angulation passes through the apex but an osteotomy is do not at a level different than the apex, the bone realigns with angulation and translation at the osteotomy site.[15,16] An example of this would be a focal dome-type osteotomy. Generally, articular deformities require osteotomy rule 2 for realignment. Rule 3 is that when osteotomy and the ACA are done at a different site than the apex of the deformity, a translational-type deformity is created.[15,16] The best example of this in the foot and ankle is a percutaneous bunion deformity. It is important to understand that when the plane of translation is the same as angulation, the apex will appear at the same level in all views; if the translation is different than the angulation, it will appear different on different views.[15,16]

Many different methods of osteotomy can be used and achieve similar outcomes. The different types that are used are opening wedges, closing wedges, displacement, step-cut, crescentic, transverse, and oblique. Transverse osteotomies are ideal for correction of rotation but are difficult to control for angular correction and often require external fixation. Closing wedge osteotomies remove a predetermined size of bone and are relatively easy. They do affect soft tissue balancing, as they often shorten the bone, but are easily fixated and often heal rapidly. Opening wedge osteotomies oppositely increase length and often need bone grafting, which can slow the healing. Oblique plan osteotomies allow for a broad surface for healing, can lengthen or shorten, and can create or correct some rotation. Focal dome osteotomies or crescentic allow for rapid healing without expense of shortening and are a great choice with the apex at the level of the joint or very close to joint. Displacement osteotomies are useful to address juxta-articular deformities, and examples of these are extension osteotomies whereby the transverse osteotomy is creased and the fragment is then rotated and the corner is impacted into the medullary canal. Step-cut osteotomies are useful for lengthening but only correct in one plane. Each osteotomy has many techniques in how to perform them and each come fraught with difficulties and complications. Practitioners must remember neurovascular bundles around the osteotomy sites, and practitioners should be cautioned when performing acute correction more than 10° unless nerve decompressions or soft tissue balancing is taken into consideration. Some are high-energy osteotomies, such as the use of a saw; some are low-energy osteotomies, such as multiple drill holes and osteotomes. Each may have advantages and disadvantages but are important in that specific instance. Osteotomies that can be done percutaneously help preserve the blood supply and allow for less scaring but require a sound understanding of anatomy bone contour as well as soft tissue overlay. High-energy osteotomies may save time but may cause thermal necrosis of the bones or delay healing and may require larger incisions. Wires can be used when preparing for wedge-type osteotomies. Mini-open techniques can be used for direct wedge osteotomies, and then percutaneous plates can be used for fixation. Other methods of fixation can be fixator-assisted platings.

The type of osteotomy can influence correction time but also fixation. Focal dome osteotomies of the ankle can be done percutaneously but only allow correction in one plane is fixed acutely. Transverse osteotomies do not provide any correction unless dynamic correction is engaged or wedge osteotomies are used.

SUMMARY

Numerous investigators and surgeons stress the importance and the technical nature of deformity planning. "Failing to plan, is planning to fail"[15] as the sensei sates in *The Art of Limb Alignment*. For treatment to be successful, whether surgical or nonsurgical, both clinical and radiographic components need to be assessed in foot and ankle deformity with consideration to proximal influence. Sound knowledge and understanding are important in attaining clinical and surgical alignment.

REFERENCES

1. Barg A, Amendola RL, Henninger HB, et al. Influence of ankle position and radiographic projection angle on measurement of supramalleolar alignment on the anteroposterior and hindfoot alignment views. Foot Ankle Int 2015;36(11):1352–61.
2. Bryant A, Tinley P, Singer K. A comparison of radiographic measurements in normal, hallux valgus, and hallux limitus feet. J Foot Ankle Surg 2000;39:39–43.
3. Engel E, Erlick N, Krems I. A simplified metatarsus adductus angle. J Am Podiatry Assoc 1983;73:620–8.
4. Fallat LM, Buckholz J. Analysis of the tailor's bunion by radiographic and anatomical display. J Am Podiatry Assoc 1980;70:597–603.
5. Fuson S, Smith S. Angular relationships of the metatarsal, talus, and calcaneus. J Am Podiatr Med Assoc 1978;68:463–6.
6. Gamble FO, Yale I. Clinical foot roentgenology. New York: Krieger Publishing Co; 1975. p. 186–208.
7. Hardy RH, Clapham JCR. Observations of hallux valgus. Based on a controlled series. J Bone Joint Surg Br 1951;33B:376–91.
8. Hass M. Radiographic and biomechanical considerations of bunion surgery. In: Gerbert J, Sokloff TH, editors. Textbook of bunion surgery. Mount Kisco (NY): Futura; 1981. p. 23–61.
9. Lamm B, Stasko PA, Gersheff M, et al. Normal foot and ankle radiographic angles, measurements, and reference points. J Foot Ankle Surg 2016;55(5):991–8.
10. LaPorta G, Melilio T, Olinski D. X-ray evaluation of hallux abducto valgus deformity. J Am Podiatry Assoc 1974;64:544–66.
11. Steel M, Johnson K, DeWitz M, et al. Radiographic measurements of the normal adult foot. Foot Ankle 1980;1:151–8.
12. Thomas J, Kunken W, Lopez R, et al. Radiographic values of the adult foot in a standardized population. J Foot Ankle Surg 2006;45(1):3–12.
13. Saltzman C, El-Khoury G. The hindfoot alignment view. Foot Ankle Int 1995;16(9):572–6.
14. Lamm BM, Paley D. Deformity correction planning for hindfoot, ankle, and lower limb. Clin Podiatr Med Surg 2004;21(3):305–26, v.
15. Standard S, Herzenberg J, Conway J, et al. The art of limb alignment. 6th edition. Rubin Institute for Advanced Orthopedics, Sinai Hospital of Baltimore; 2017.
16. Paley D, Herzenberg J. Principles of deformity correction. 1st edition. Springer; 2002.

Current Advancements in Ankle Arthrodiastasis

Jacob Wynes, DPM, MS[a],*, Andreas C. Kaikis, DPM[b]

KEYWORDS

- Ankle distraction • Ankle arthritis • Ilizarov • Supramalleolar osteotomy
- External fixation • Arthrodiastasis

KEY POINTS

- Ankle arthrodiastasis allows the clinician to follow a continuum of care before commitment to joint destruction procedures, such as ankle implant arthroplasty or fusion.
- The optimal distance for distraction should exceed 5 mm to withstand axial loading force during weightbearing.
- The application of hinged distraction with the use of Ilizarov hinges, in line with Inman's axis, allows for optimal modulation of ankle hydrostatic pressure and nourishment to the articular cartilage during distraction.
- Physiologic changes have been shown to occur at the cellular level in response to ankle distraction, which assists in diminishing subchondral sclerosis and pain from end-stage ankle arthritis.
- Simultaneous deformity correction is a viable option and should be considered in the setting of posttraumatic ankle arthritis.

INTRODUCTION

The devastating sequelae of ankle arthritis is comparable to hip arthritis and end-stage heart failure in quality-of-life measurements.[1,2] Most instances of ankle osteoarthritis develop after inciting traumatic events and affect both the pediatric and adult population.[3–5] Patients with posttraumatic arthritis tend to be younger, with joint preservation techniques shown to be desirable in improving overall lifestyle.[6] Options such as arthrodesis are effective, but will result in compensation and often adjacent joint arthrosis, particularly with cases of malunion.[7]

The term arthrodiastasis was formulated by the word stems of arthro (joint), dia (through), and tasis (to stretch out) by Aldegheri and colleagues[8] from Verona, Italy. Volkov and Oganesian[9] in 1975 performed the first hinged distraction of the elbow and knee and demonstrated it to be a viable treatment option. A few years later Judet

Disclosure Statement: Consultant Orthofix (J. Wynes). No disclosures (A.C. Kaikis).
[a] Department of Orthopaedics, University of Maryland School of Medicine, Baltimore, MD 21043, USA; [b] Department of Podiatric Surgery, University of Pennsylvania, Penn Presbyterian Medical Center, 51 N. 39th Street, Philadelphia, PA 19104, USA
* Corresponding author. 4110 Tall Willows Road, Ellicott City, MD 21043.
E-mail address: jwynes@som.umaryland.edu

and Judet[10] in 1978 performed the first hinged distraction of the ankle joint and proved it to be a viable method to achieve joint separation and maintenance of anatomic motion. Increased popularity in Europe was gained from work by Marijnissen and associates with their work showing benefits of distraction in the treatment of end-stage osteoarthritis within the ankle joint.[11]

The treatment of ankle joint osteoarthritis continues to evolve with innovation in joint-sparing and joint-destructive interventions. Ankle arthrodiastasis continues to be a viable treatment option to decrease pain and increase function in the younger patient with ankle osteoarthritis while preserving the native ankle joint. In this article, we aim to review contemporary perspectives on arthrodiastasis of the ankle and present a case reports illustrating these concepts.

HYPOTHESIS/RATIONALE

The rationale behind arthrodiastasis is a continuous, reparative process to counteract the destruction of native, articular cartilage.[11] The procedure involves weightbearing with an external fixator to place traction across the joint space. It is speculated that mechanical unloading through distraction allows for chondrocytes to repair in the intermittent intraarticular fluid pressure environment.[12] Additionally, stress shielding occurs, which allows for subchondral cyst resorption and less subchondral bone sclerosis.[11] Fibrocartilage is formed during the distraction process, which seals the cartilage to the cystic area and eliminates synovial fluid of cysts, thus decreasing pain.[11] It is also hypothesized that arthrodiastasis has an effect on decreasing the arthritic impetus in the ankle joint by on an unknown effect of proteoglycans.[12] These benefits alleviate stiffness within the joint and improve motion and pain for the patient.

Arthrodiastasis is a surgical technique used to promote morphoangiogenesis and serves to decrease subchondral sclerosis adjacent to joint surfaces through stress shielding. Nociceptive fibers are located within the joint capsule, ligaments, periosteum, and subchondral bone.[13] Distraction allows for decreasing intraarticular pressure and thereby diminishes the nociceptive influence. Additionally, control of the catabolic environment and oxidized stress to chondrocytes by unloading the joint surface and regulation of the cytokine cascade creates regenerative effects to osteochondral damage.[14–16]

INDICATIONS

The ideal surgical candidate for ankle arthrodiastasis is often less than 50 years of age and presents with isolated unilateral primary or posttraumatic osteoarthritis of the ankle. Ankle joint plain film radiographs and further workup in the form of a computed tomography scan assesses the amount of joint space involved. It is not uncommon to visualize ankle joint narrowing from an anteroposterior or mortise view, yet the joint space is often maintained on a true lateral view (**Fig. 1**). These patients would benefit most from a supplemental ankle arthrotomy and adjunctive tibial and talar exostectomy. Further patient considerations include pain that is disabling and failure with offloading strategies to include rocker bottom shoes, injections, and other forms of conservative therapy. Numerous reports have demonstrated efficacy with hip avascular necrosis in pathology such as Legg-Calvé-Perthes, which could be implemented in the management of talar avascular necrosis as well.[17]

CONTRAINDICATIONS

At this time, based on thorough gleaning of the literature the authors do not believe there to be a body mass index cutoff for surgical arthrodiastasis. However, patients

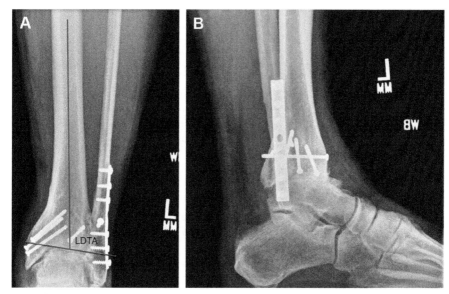

Fig. 1. (*A*, *B*) Preoperative radiographic assessment anteroposterior and lateral projections demonstrating decreased joint space varus malalignment and ankle boney ectopy and impingement anteriorly. Note the lateral distal tibial angle (LDTA) of 102° and anterior distal tibial angle of 86°.

who are poor candidates for application of external fixation, such as those with lymphedema or prone to volume overload or swelling, should be excluded. Additionally, patients who present with a diagnosis of inflammatory arthritis, fibromyalgia, chronic regional pain syndrome, neuropathy/neuroarthropathy, suspicion for septic arthritis/osteomyelitis, or inability to follow-up for routine evaluation should be considered for other treatment options. All other factors may be left to the surgeon's discretion.[11,14]

RECENT COMPARISONS OF PREOPERATIVE AND POSTOPERATIVE PARAMETERS

Intema and colleagues[18] evaluated the subchondral bone density of individuals via computed tomography scanning. In their prospective study, patients received dual-contrast computed tomography scans performed preoperatively and at 1 and 2 years postoperatively. Each patient underwent ankle arthrodiastasis with an Ilizarov frame for 3 months. Their study demonstrated pain relief and functional improvement in all patients. Imaging demonstrated decreases in subchondral bone density at 1-year and 2-year imaging in accordance with measurements in bone density per Hounsfield unit.

Lamm and colleagues[19] also performed a preoperative and postoperative imaging study for 3 patients who underwent hinged ankle distraction for 4 months. The average age of the patients was 41 years Preoperative and postoperative T1- and T2-weighted sagittal and coronal MRIs were collected from 3 patients. On the preoperative and postoperative MRIs, the subchondral bone of the tibiotalar joint, cartilage, thickness or joint space and number of subchondral cysts of the joints were measured. Postoperative MRI scans performed an average 13 months after surgery demonstrated subchondral bone thickness decreased by 0.5 mm, the average postoperative cartilage thickness or joint space increased by an average of 0.5 mm, and the average subchondral bone cysts of the talus and tibia decreased in number and size.

SURGICAL ADVANCES AND INNOVATIONS WITH ANKLE ARTHRODIASTASIS

The outlined tables demonstrate aspects of arthrodiastasis that the authors deem necessary to truly unlock the value of the procedure. They paucity of the literature related to these aspects of arthrodiastasis indicates there should be further investigation into them (**Fig. 2**).

Although it may be intuitive to perform and scantly documented in literature, the concomitant procedure of performing an adjunctive tibiotalar exostectomy is of importance in arthrodiastasis. To free the joint of impinging osteophytes, an exostectomy is valuable in helping to achieve the goal of increasing the ankle range of motion (**Table 1**).

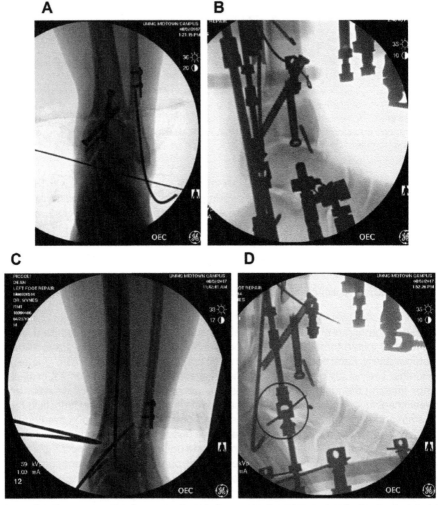

Fig. 2. (*A*, *B*) Intraoperative fluoroscopic view demonstrating placement of axis wire (red circle) in keeping with Inman's axis to maintain anatomic range of motion at the ankle joint complex on the anteroposterior and lateral views. (*C*) Completion of supramalleolar osteotomy with provisional fixation. (*D*) Lateral view demonstrating acute distraction of 5 mm intraoperatively.

Table 1		
Adjunctive tibiotalar exostectomy		
Study Design	**No. of Patients**	**Recommendations/Outcome**
Retrospective case series	25/32	Consideration with osseous equinus deformity

The authors believe that this is performed more frequently than cited in the literature based on review of the literature, particularly, if an open ankle arthrodiastasis is performed.

Data from Paley D, Lamm B, Purohit RM, et al. Distraction arthroplasty of the ankle-how far can you stretch the indications? Foot Ankle Clin N Am 2008;13:471–84.

Paley and colleagues[20] in their retrospective case series of patients who underwent arthrodiastasis highlighted their adjunctive surgical procedures. Twenty-five patients underwent anterior ankle osteophyte resections and 3 patients underwent posterior ankle osteophyte resections. The authors postulate that the addition of a tibiotalar exostectomy is valuable in allowing the acute and gradual distraction of the joint as well of removing any obvious detriment to the range of motion of the ankle.

Van Valburg and colleagues[21] were among the first to investigate the amount of distraction necessary to allow for successful arthrodiastasis. In their 1995 research, they observed that a distraction of 5.0 mm gradually (0.5 mm twice daily for 5 days) starting on postoperative day 1 yielded positive results in their patients. They reported that 55% of the patients had increased ankle range of motion and joint width widening. This was the first documented measurement recommendation for distraction (**Table 2**).

Table 2					
Amount of intraarticular distraction					
Study Type	**Sample Size**	**Gender**	**Ages (y)**	**Follow-up**	**Recommendations/ Outcome**
Retrospective case series	11	7 male/4 female	35 ± 13	20 mo ± 6 mo.	Patients had decreased pain with 5 pain free, range of motion increased 55%, joint width widening in 55%, recommend 5.0 mm of distraction gap
Cadaveric	9	3 male/6 female	39–60; mean 55	N/A	At 700 N of load there must be 5.8 mm of distraction gap for no contact of the tibiotalar joint during weightbearing; 7.0 on nonweightbearing radiography

Data from van Valburg AA, van Roermund P, Lammens J, et al. Can Ilizarov joint distraction delay the need for an arthrodesis of the ankle? A preliminary report. J Bone Joint Surg Br 1995;77–B(5):720–5; and Fragomen A, McCoy T, Meyers L, et al. Minimum distraction gap: how much ankle joint space is enough in ankle distraction arthroplasty? HSS J 2013;10(1):6–12.

Fragomen and colleagues[3] later studied the amount of distraction through the use cadaveric specimens. They defined the minimum distraction gap as the space that was created iatrogenically in the joint by distracting it with the fixator. After applying circular frames to 9 cadaveric specimens, they applied various loads of force and then measured radiographic joint space and joint contact pressure. Their results created the "minimum distraction gap" that would provide unloading of the tibiotalar joint at 700 N. They postulated that a distraction gap of 5.8 mm would allow no contact during full weightbearing through the external fixator (**Table 3**).

The authors agree that adequate distraction is necessary to unload the tibiotalar joint and provide the ideal environment for cartilaginous repair. Weightbearing through the apparatus is of utmost importance and must be maintained by the fixation and adjunctive foot plate (**Fig. 3**). The authors believe that the original 5 mm of acute distraction postulated by Van Valburg and colleagues allows for appropriate joint mechanical offloading and resistance to cyclical axial load. The authors additionally provide 5 mm of gradual distraction to allow for desensitization of the nociceptive influence within the joint capsule and modulation of hydrostatic pressure.

As ankle arthrodiastasis becomes more common in practice, the procedure undergoes various modifications. Paley and colleagues[20] were the first to publish on the use of hinged distraction versus static Ilizarov distraction. They postulated that the hinged distractor allowed for range of motion exercises. To allow the hinge the function appropriately, they performed soft tissue releases and exostectomy as needed. In their retrospective series of 18 patients, 11 reported satisfaction with the procedure and 2 patients required total ankle arthroplasty or fusion (**Fig. 4**).

In 2012, Saltzman and colleagues[22] performed a prospective investigation of motion-distracted frames and static frames. In their study of 36 patients that were randomly assigned, patients had the fixator on for 3 months. The observations of the study yielded better ankle osteoarthritis scale scores of the motion-distracted frames at 26, 52, and 104 weeks over the static frames. Overall they illustrated that adjunctive ankle dorsiflexion and plantarflexion showed both an early and sustained benefit to the procedure.

Yang and colleagues[23] published their study in 2017 in which all their patients underwent a documented hinged distraction for 3 months. The mean American Orthopedic Foot and Ankle Society Score scores, Short Form-36 scores, and visual analog scale scores improved moderately. The authors reported that one patient went on to ankle fusion at 1 year and one at 3 years postoperatively. The authors' preferred method is to use a hinged distractor to allow for mobilization of the joint.

Posttraumatic arthritis is usually the inciting factor in most of the ankle pain that foot and ankle surgeon witnesses in the postulation. Rotational ankle fractures and distal tibial fractures are often detrimental to the structural integrity of the tibiotalar joint. The nonoperative treatment of the these fractures as well as open reduction internal fixation can lead to malposition of the joint. To allow for the joint to benefit from arthrodiastasis, the authors find it necessary in cases to perform a supramalleolar osteotomy. This step allows for better positioning of the joint and distraction can be performed to enhance the joint environment through reduction in shear forces and decreasing uneven contact area (**Fig. 5**).

Stapleton and Zgonis[4] described a case of arthrodiastasis and supramalleolar osteotomy of a 16-year-old girl. With the presenting posttraumatic valgus deformity, the authors performed a focal dome osteotomy and fibular osteotomy to realign the joint. They placed the ankle in 5° to 7° of recurvatum with slight posterior translation to correct for the valgus deformity. After fixating the osteotomy with a 6.5-mm cannulated screw, they performed ankle distraction for 3 months. The authors reported

Table 3 Adjunctive hinged distraction and passive range of motion					
Study Type	Sample Size	Gender	Age (y)	Follow-up	Outcome
Retrospective	18	7 Male/11 Female	45; range 17–62	Mean, 64 mo; range, 24–157 mo	Mean foot and ankle questionnaire 71/100 (range, 44–98) Mean foot and ankle questionnaire shoe comfort 47/100 (range, 0–100) 4/18 used assisted device for ambulation 2/18 went on to fusion/TAR 11/18 very satisfied or satisfied with surgery
Prospective	36	Fixed 11 male/7 female	42.8 (range, 18–53)	104 wk	Motion-distraction group had significantly better AOS scores than fixed at 26, 52, and 104 wk after frame removal
		Motion 13 male/5 female	42.7 (range, 27–59)	104 wk	At 104 wk motion group had improvement of 56.65 in AOS score vs fixed of 22.9%
Retrospective	16	6 male/10 female	30.3 ± 14.3 (range, 14–60)	mean 40.9 mo ± 14.7 (range, 16–67 mo)	VAS improved from 5.9 ± 0.8–3.7 ± 2.2 ($P = .0028$) Mean AOFAS score improved from 41.9 ± 7.2 to 68.1 ± 20.0 ($P = .001$) Mean SF-36 score improved from 43.1 ± 7.6 to 62.7 ± 18.8 ($P = .002$) 1/16 onto ankle fusion at 1 yr, 1/16 at 3 y Overall 9/16 reported benefits at 41 mo

Abbreviations: AOFAS, American Orthopedic Foot and Ankle Society Score; AOS, Ankle Osteoarthritis Scale; SF-36, Short Form 36; TAR, total ankle replacement; VAS, visual analog scale.
    Data from Refs.[20,22,23]

healed osteotomies at 6 months with improved function, decreased pain, and increased range of motion at 22 months (**Table 4**).
    Zhao and colleagues[24] published on the correction of a varus posttraumatic ankle of a 57-year-old woman using supramalleolar osteotomy with arthrodiastasis for

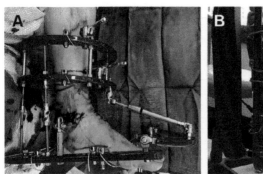
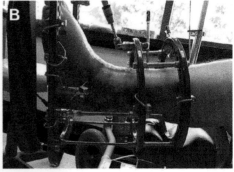
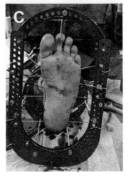

Fig. 3. (*A, B*) Clinical photographs of the foot and ankle perioperatively. Note the hinge placement medial and lateral as well as the dynamic strut, which allows dorsiflexion and plantarflexion. (*C*) Clinical intraoperative photograph depicting wire placement before foot plate application.

3 months. The authors used a medial opening wedge osteotomy with fibular osteotomy with plating. The authors reported bony union of the osteotomies at 4 months. The patient was followed 3 years postoperatively with an increased American Orthopedic Foot and Ankle Society Score from 26 to 85 and the space enlargement from distraction was maintained.

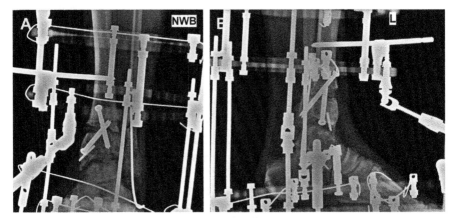

Fig. 4. (*A, B*) Anteroposterior and lateral plain film radiographs demonstrating maintenance of joint space with external fixator and obtaining 10 mm of desired distraction. A lateral distal tibial angle of 90° obtained and restoration of an anterior distal tibial angle of 80°.

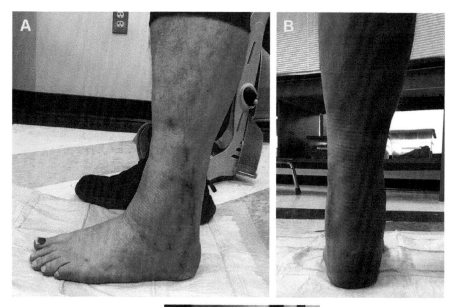

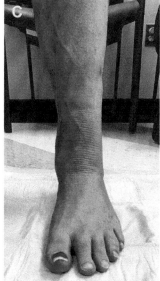

Fig. 5. Clinical photographs of the patient 9 months status post external fixator removal (and 1 year status post index procedure). (*A*) Lateral, (*B*) posterior (*C*) anterior views post external fixator removal.

The authors' value the use of supramalleolar osteotomies as adjunct procedures for ankle arthrodiastasis for the malpositioned ankle, particularly with varus deformity. Evaluation of the mechanical axis deviation and resolving the deformity apex using erect long leg standing views can also aid the clinician in elucidating where the deformity lies. In posttraumatic deformity, biplanar deformity should always be suspected because ankle fractures often predispose to the apex at the level of the ankle joint itself, whereas congenital deformity often presents proximal to the

	Sample		Age	Follow-up	
Study Type	Size	Gender	(y)	(mo)	Outcome
Case report	1	Female	16	22	Healed osteotomies at 6 mo; improved function, increased range of motion, diminished pain
Case report	1	Female	57	36	Healed osteotomies at 4 mo; AOFAS score increased from 26 to 85, ankle dorsiflexion from 10° to 24°

Table 4
Adjunctive supramalleolar tibial osteotomy

Abbreviation: AOFAS, American Orthopedic Foot and Ankle Society Score.
  Data from Stapleton J, Zgonis T. Supramalleolar osteotomy and ankle arthrodiastasis for juvenile posttraumatic ankle arthritis. Clin Podiatr Med Surg 2014;31:597–601; and Zhao HM, Liang XJ, Li Y, et al. Supramalleolar osteotomy with distraction arthroplasty in treatment of varus ankle osteoarthritis with large talar tilt angle: a case report and literature review. J Foot Ankle Surg 2017;56(5):1125–8.

joint. The disadvantage of concomitant supramalleolar osteotomy is sometimes increasing the amount of time in the external fixator while awaiting healing of the osteotomies.

POSTOPERATIVE COURSE

Postoperatively, the patient is permitted to bear weight immediately after their surgical procedure. Acute distraction of the ankle joint is performed in the operating room of 5 mm and after 5 days of elevation the patient is instructed to distract the ankle 1 mm/d or 4 one-quarter turns along the distraction/threaded rod. A maximal length of 10 mm is achieved and once the swelling has dissipated over the course of 1 to 2 weeks, the authors recommend hinged distraction twice a day for 20 repetitions. The external fixator is maintained with "pin care" consisting of 2% chlorhexidine wipes along the fixator with changes of the gauze surrounding the pin sites twice per week. Serial radiographic radiographs are obtained at 4-week intervals barring any acute issues requiring images, such as suspicion for pin lucency. The radiographic assessment is used to assess ankle distraction and the dissipation of subchondral sclerosis at the joint interface. The fixator is maintained for a goal of 3 months in accordance with published studies.

CASE REPORT

We present the case of an active 56-year-old man with a notable past medical history of hypertension, anxiety, and a 10-year history of prior trimalleolar ankle fracture to his left ankle. His ankle pain continued to worsen and he presented to the office with an inability to maintain activity secondary to swelling and pain. The patient was offered joint-sparing options to include ankle arthrodiastasis and total ankle arthroplasty, and the joint-destructive procedure of ankle arthrodesis. After discussion, he elected to proceed with removal of hardware, focal dome osteotomy of the supramalleolar region, and hinged ankle arthrodiastasis. This decision was based on an in-depth discussion with the patient reviewing the risks and alternatives and likely equivocal longevity with distraction as opposed to ankle replacement (**Fig. 6**).

The patient underwent the surgery as described herein with inclusion of a tibial exostectomy as an adjunct. Serial radiographs were followed to assess healing of the

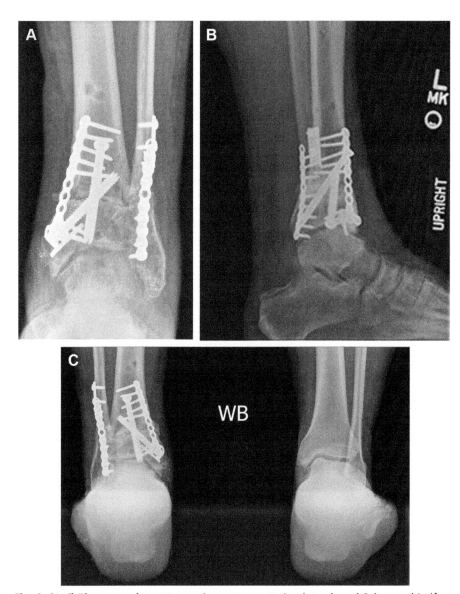

Fig. 6. (A–C) Three months postoperative anteroposterior, lateral, and Saltzman hindfoot axial radiographs status post fixator removal with autogenous calcaneal bone grafting and plating of the tibia medial and fibula posteriorly.

supramalleolar osteotomy, and visualization of morphoangiogenesis/osteopenia and decreased subchondral sclerosis. At 3 months, the patient was scheduled for removal of the external fixator with adjunctive bone graft application and plating of the medial distal tibia and posterior fibula to assist in healing the supramalleolar osteotomy. Of note, the patient was able to bear weight in his external fixator throughout the entire perioperative process. At 9 months status post external fixator removal, the patient is out of his controlled ankle motion walker boot and participates in further strengthening and range of motion exercises to his ankle and subtalar joint complex with the aid of physical therapy.

SUMMARY

As this case illustrates, when combining supramalleolar osteotomy with hinged ankle arthrodiastasis, care must be taken to ensure appropriate wire configuration and recognition of the axis of hinge placement, because this could impact the unique dynamic nature of this treatment regimen. Additionally, one should pay attention to micromotion at the osteotomy, which is subtle. This motion may create mild instability, particularly as distraction of the ankle is also occurring. Incorporation of an Ilizarov-style circular frame with hinged distraction and encouragement of passive range of motion further provides an environment for cartilage regeneration.[25] End-stage osteoarthritis of the ankle is amenable to arthrodiastasis by achieving symptomatic relief and restoring pain-free motion without burning the proverbial "bridge" of needing an ankle fusion or replacement in the future as innovation in these techniques advance.

REFERENCES

1. Glazebrook M, Daniels T, Younger A, et al. Comparison of health related quality of life between patients with end-stage ankle and hip arthrosis. J Bone Joint Surg Am 2008;90:499–505.

2. Zaidi R, Pfeil M, Macgregor A, et al. How do patients with end-stage ankle arthritis decided between two surgical treatments? A qualitative study. BMJ Open 2013; 3(7) [pii:e002782].

3. Fragomen A, McCoy T, Meyers L, et al. Minimum distraction gap: how much ankle joint space is enough in ankle distraction arthroplasty? HSS J 2013;10(1):6–12.

4. Stapleton J, Zgonis T. Supramalleolar osteotomy and ankle arthrodiastasis for juvenile posttraumatic ankle arthritis. Clin Podiatr Med Surg 2014;31:597–601.

5. Tellisi N, Fragomen AT, Kleinman D, et al. Joint preservation of the osteoarthritic ankle using distraction arthroplasty. Foot Ankle Int 2009;30(4):318–25.

6. DiDomenico L, Gatalyak N. End-stage ankle arthritis. Clin Podiatr Med Surg 2012; 29:391–5.

7. Fuchs S, Sandman C, Skwara A, et al. Quality of life 20 years after arthrodesis of the ankle: a study of adjacent joints. J Bone Joint Surg Br 2003;85(7):994–8.

8. Aldegheri R, Trivella G, Saleh M. Articulated distraction of the hip: conservative surgery for arthritis in young patients. Clin Orthop Relat Res 1994;301:94–101.

9. Volkov MV, Oganesian OV. Restoration of function in the knee and elbow with a hinge-distractor apparatus. J Bone Joint Surg Am 1975;57(5):591–600.

10. Judet R, Judet T. The use of hinge distraction apparatus after arthrolysis and arthroplasty (author's transl). Rev Chir Orthop Reparatrice Appar Mot 1978;64(5): 353–65 [in French].

11. Maijnissen AC, van Roermund PM, Verzijl N, et al. Does joint distraction result in actual repair of cartilage in experimentally induced osteoarthritis? Arthritis Rheum 2001;44:S306.

12. Marijnissen AC, Vincken KL, Viergever MA. Ankle images digital analysis: digital measurement of joint space width and subchondral sclerosis on standard radiographs. Osteoarthritis Cartilage 2004;9:264–72.

13. Stauffer R, Chao EY, Brewster RC. Force and motion analysis of the normal, diseased and prosthetic ankle joint. Clin Orthop Relat Res 1997;127:189–96.

14. Marijnissen AC, van Roermund P, Van Melkebeek J, et al. Clinical benefit of joint distraction in the treatment of severe osteoarthritis of the ankle: proof of concept in an open prospective study and randomized controlled study. Arthritis Rheum 2002;46(11):2893–902.
15. van Valburg AA, van Roermund PM, Marijnissen AC, et al. Joint distraction in treatment of osteoarthritis: a two year follow-up of the ankle. Osteoarthritis Cartilage 1999;7(5):474–9.
16. Castagnini F, Pellegrini C, Perazzo L, et al. Joint sparing treatments in early ankle osteoarthritis: current procedures and future perspectives. J Exp Orthop 2016; 3(1):3.
17. Laklouk MA, Hosny GA. Hinged distraction of the hip joint in the treatment of Perthes disease: evaluation at skeletal maturity. J Pediatr Orthop B 2012;21(5): 386–93.
18. Intema F, Thomas TP, Anderson DD, et al. Subchondral bone remodeling is related to clinical improvement after joint distraction in the treatment of ankle osteoarthritis. Osteoarthritis Cartilage 2011;19(6):668–75.
19. Lamm B, Gourdine-Shaw M. MRI evaluation of ankle distraction: a preliminary report. Clin Podiatr Med Surg 2009;26(2):185–91.
20. Paley D, Lamm B, Purohit RM, et al. Distraction arthroplasty of the ankle-how far can you stretch the indications? Foot Ankle Clin 2008;13:471–84.
21. van Valburg AA, van Roermund P, Lammens J, et al. Can Ilizarov joint distraction delay the need for an arthrodesis of the ankle? A preliminary report. J Bone Joint Surg Br 1995;77-B(5):720–5.
22. Saltzman CL, Hills SL, Stolley MP, et al. Motion versus fixed distraction of the joint in the treatment of ankle osteoarthritis: a prospective randomized controlled trial. J Bone Joint Surg Am 2012;94(11):961–70.
23. Yang X, Yuan X, Xu XY. Ankle joint distraction arthroplasty for severe ankle arthritis. BMC Musculoskelet Disord 2018;18(1):1–7.
24. Zhao HM, Liang XJ, Li Y, et al. Supramalleolar osteotomy with distraction arthroplasty in treatment of varus ankle osteoarthritis with large talar tilt angle: a case report and literature review. J Foot Ankle Surg 2017;56(5):1125–8.
25. van Valburg AA, van Roy HL, Lafeber FP, et al. Beneficial effects of intermittent fluid pressure of low physiologic magnitude on cartilage and inflammation in osteoarthritis. An in vitro study. J Rheumatol 1998;25(3):515–20.

The Gradual and Acute Correction of Equinus Using External Fixation

Michael Subik, DPM[a,b,*], Mark Shearer, DPM, ACFAS[b,c],
Ali M. Saleh, DPM, BA[a], Guido A. LaPorta, DPM, MS[d,e]

KEYWORDS

- Equinus • External fixation • Ilizarov • Acute correction • Gradual correction
- Hexapod • Buttress frame

KEY POINTS

- Owing to the variability of diagnostic parameters of equinus, this article serves to review the proper clinical workup and identification of the deformity.
- This article reviews the literature, highlighting surgical treatment options for the management of varying pathologies that have an equinus deformity as one of their components.
- Discussion and review of the author's technique and use of external fixation for the correction of equinus deformity, either gradually or acutely, will be concentrated on.

INTRODUCTION

It is well-known that equinus deformity has been related to a multitude of lower extremity pathologies. These include but are not limited to Achilles tendinopathy, posterior tibial tendonitis, pes planus, plantar fasciitis, Lisfranc arthrosis, Charcot neuroarthropathy, hallux valgus, and hallux limitus.[1–3] Equinus is defined simply as insufficient ankle joint dorsiflexion for normal gait, resulting in lower extremity compensation, pathology, or a combination of both with normal gait requiring more than 10° of dorsiflexion with the knee extended.[1]

Equinus is something that has previously been associated with spastic and neurologically impaired individuals with little attention being paid to the more subtle contractures.[2] The manifestations of equinus, previously overlooked, underdiagnosed, or undertreated, are frequently more recognized and have garnered more attention.[2,4,5]

[a] Northern New Jersey Reconstructive Foot and Ankle, St. Mary's General Hospital, Podiatric Residency, 350 Boulevard, Passaic, NJ 07055, USA; [b] Northern New Jersey Reconstructive Foot and Ankle Fellowship, 160 Ridge Road, Lyndhurst, NJ 07071, USA; [c] Residency Training, Our Lady of Lourdes Memorial Hospital, 169 Riverside Drive, Binghamton, NY 13905, USA; [d] Geisinger Community Medical Center, 1800 Mulberry Street, Scranton, PA 18510, USA; [e] Our Lady of Lourdes Memorial Hospital, 169 Riverside Drive, Binghamton, NY 13905, USA
* Corresponding author. Northern New Jersey Reconstructive Foot and Ankle, St. Mary's General Hospital, 350 Boulevard, Passaic, NJ 07055.
E-mail address: drsubik@gmail.com

Clin Podiatr Med Surg 35 (2018) 481–496
https://doi.org/10.1016/j.cpm.2018.05.007
0891-8422/18/© 2018 Elsevier Inc. All rights reserved.

podiatric.theclinics.com

Numerous nonoperative and operative treatment options have been published and researched to varying degrees of success. When it comes to the more severe forms of equinus caused by trauma, burn contractures, and neurologic deficits, standard surgical interventions, which include open soft tissue releases, tendon transfers, osteotomies, and arthrodeses alone, do not suffice for the restoration of normal ankle joint range of motion because these procedures are often associated with more soft tissue and neurovascular complications. It is at that point that further means of addressing the deformity, through the use of gradual correction of external fixation, is required.

The goal of this article is to provide the foot and ankle surgeon with an overview of the equinus itself with a brief discussion about the clinical classification and identification of the deformity. However, it also serves to provide an insight on the various treatment methods for the deformity, specifically concentrating on the use of external fixation in a variety of techniques to correct the deformity, either acutely or gradually, increasing the physician's surgical armamentarium.

BIOMECHANICAL COMPENSATION

Literature remarks, "the worst foot in the world is the one with a fully compensated equinus deformity."[6] The compensation for equinus includes rearfoot pronation, hypermobile flatfoot, early heel-off, and an abducted gait pattern.[3] The gastrocsoleus complex is the most significant medial arch flattening structure of the lower extremity. A tight gastrocsoleus leads to subtalar joint pronation, which evolves into eventual frontal plane eversion of the medial column, decreasing the lever arm of peroneus longus, resulting in dorsiflexion of the first metatarsal and cuneiform, and plantarflexion of the navicular and talus.[6]

Additionally, the body's center of gravity is displaced posteriorly when there is a restriction of dorsiflexion at the ankle joint, to which the body compensates by adjusting the motion that occurs at adjacent joints, not only distal to, but also proximal to the restricted ankle joint to realign the center of gravity. Proximal compensations such as genu recurvatum, and also lumbar lordosis with hip and knee flexion facilitate a forward shift of the body's center of gravity. These conditions can, however, lead to major pathologies, such as knee dysfunction and chronic low back pain.[1,7-9]

Distal compensation results when a tight gastrocsoleus complex does not allow the required 8° to 10° of ankle joint dorsiflexion for normal anterior advancement of the tibia over the foot during midstance.[6]

CLASSIFICATION AND CAUSES

Equinus is defined as the inability to dorsiflex the ankle enough to allow the heel to contact the supporting surface without some form of biomechanical compensation. In the pediatric population, equinus is associated with a variety of congenital deformities, such as Charcot-Marie-Tooth disease, cerebral palsy, spina bifida, myelomeningocoele, muscular dystrophy, arthrogryposis, fibular hemimelia, clubfoot, and limb length discrepancy. Equinus can be a consequence of poliomyelitis, trauma, burns, and limb lengthening procedures. Immobilization after trauma, lack of function of the involved limb, or compensation for other conditions can be causes of equinus in adults.[10]

At present, there is a general lack of consensus with regard to the correlation of the diagnosis and initiation of absolute treatment of equinus because the actual magnitude of reduction in range of motion required predisposing to lower limb abnormalities is unknown. As such, Charles and colleagues[11] developed a 2-stage definition system for equinus that relates these 2 factors. Stage 1 is defined as dorsiflexion of less than 10°, indicating minor compensation and minor increased forefoot pressure. Stage 2 is a reflection of dorsiflexion of less than 5°, which translates to major compensatory changes leading to major increased forefoot pressure. This system has, therefore, been shown to assist in the standardization of the diagnosis of the deformity in the absence of definitive data.

Barouk and Barouk[12] refer to Digiovanni's study where 2 types of short gastocnemius are quantitatively defined: first, ankle dorsiflexion equal or inferior to 110° and/ or a differential average of 11.3° between a straight and a flexed knee.

The classification of ankle joint equinus can be categorized into muscular (gastrocnemius/gastrocsoleus), osseous, and combination forms, which can be further subdivided into spastic and nonspastic.[5,13] Two other causes of equinus that merit a brief discussion is aging and type 2 diabetes. Grimston and colleagues[14] found that, when comparing ankle joint range of motion in young and old male and female volunteers, the latter were found to have 29% less ankle joint range of motion than the former, which most likely is due to increased elastic stiffness.[11]

Additionally, with type 2 diabetes mellitus, the association of increased oxidative stress and increased glycation of proteins found in this disease has been linked to being a possible contributing factor to a decrease in joint range of motion.[11,15,16] Studies have shown that glycation of connective tissue proteins induces structural changes within tendons, contributing to the shortening of muscles and a decrease in their compliance.[11,17,18]

CLINICAL WORKUP

The Silfverskiöld test helps in differentiating between gastrocnemius and gastrocsoleus equinus. The clinician places the patient in a supine position and ankle joint dorsiflexion is assessed and compared with the knee in extension and in flexion. In isolated gastrocnemius equinus, the range of motion at the ankle joint is increased with the knee bent at 90°, essentially eliminating restrictive influences from the gastrocnemius muscle. Barouk and Barouk[12] found that, in isolated gastrocnemius equinus, there is a difference of at least 13° of increased ankle joint dorsiflexion with the knee bent compared with the knee fully extended. If there is no difference in the ankle range of motion with the knee extended or flexed, this finding may indicate a gastrocsoleus equinus. In this situation, if the clinician deems the restriction of the ankle joint comes to an abrupt stop upon dorsiflexion, an osseous equinus would then have to be ruled out through further imaging.[5,13]

DiGiovanni and colleagues[19] have challenged the idea of diagnosing ankle equinus solely through physical examination as clinicians are not perfect using a clinical examination. Potential sources of error include the knee position, the position in which the patient is being examined, the configuration of the subtalar joint during assessment, incorrect placement of the goniometer against the lower extremity when used, and so on.[11,20,21] The clinician can decrease these chances of error by ensuring that the patient does not contract the extensors, the dorsiflexory moment exerted is not greater than 2 kg of force, and that the hindfoot is reduced away from valgus to a more neutral or varus position.[12] An 8.5° to 10.0° difference has been found when measuring equinus in the foot when comparing a supinated foot with a pronated foot. Placing the foot in the maximally supinated position when clinically assessing the ankle joint locks the midtarsal joint to 2.5°, essentially allowing for a less variable measurement of ankle joint dorsiflexion.[22]

RADIOGRAPHIC FINDINGS IN EQUINUS

Equinus is measured by the tibial-sole angle, which is measured by drawing a line along the sole (ie, plantar aspect of the first metatarsal head to the plantar calcaneus) and join it with a line along the long axis of the tibia. Equinus is the amount of uncorrectable plantarflexion from neutral (tibial-sole angle >90°). Mild is considered to be less than 20° from neutral, moderate 20° to 40° from neutral, and severe being greater than 40° from neutral.[23] Some of the radiographic findings in equinus include decreased calcaneal inclination angle, increased talocalcaneal angle, and increased talar declination angle (**Fig. 1**). Owing to the contribution of midfoot equinus to global foot equinus being underappreciated, Elomrani and colleagues[24] developed a new radiographic technique, the lateral mid tibia to toes weightbearing view of the foot and ankle, which was a method of assessing both ankle and midfoot equinus.

TREATMENT

Treatment options for equinus can range from conservative measures to more intricate surgical interventions, involving soft tissue and osseous structures. If the primary etiology is of soft tissue in origin, conservative instructions are often given initially to begin a rigorous regimen of stretching exercises to increase dorsiflexion at the ankle joint. Studies have shown, however, that there is an improvement of only a few degrees after different levels and times of stretching of the gastrocnemius muscle.[4,25,26] Furthermore, Barrett questions even the need for stretching the muscle or aponeurosis, because the tensile strength that would be required to stretch the aponeurosis would far exceed the force required to maintain normal ligamentous and tendon integrity of the midfoot during the stretch.[4,27] Other conservative treatment options include dynamic splinting and serial casting, which are appropriately attempted for the management of mild equinus deformities.[28]

After conservative therapy fails, surgical treatment options are explored. For nonspastic gastrocnemius equinus, which is considered to be the most common etiologic type of ankle equinus, distal recession of the gastrocnemius aponeurosis is a viable option owing to its association with less disability and fewer complications.[5] Furthermore, there are some who advocate performing a gastrocnemius recession as the primary procedure when surgically addressing complex forefoot deformities. With equinus being linked to a plethora of pathologies, the rationale behind primarily

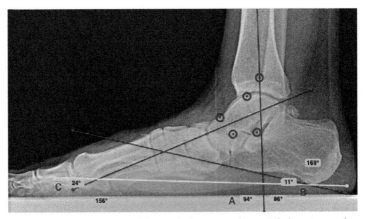

Fig. 1. (A) Tibial sole angle measured by angle between the weightbearing surface and the tibial bisector—normal neutral. (B) Calcaneal inclination angle measured by angle between the weightbearing surface and the plantar calcaneal cortex—normal is approximately 20°. (C) Talar declination angle measured by angle between the weightbearing surface and the bisector of body/neck of talus—normal is approximately 21°.

performing a gastrocnemius recession is that it decreases the actual number of surgical procedures required and often completely eliminates the need for a second surgery. Barrett[4] has found forefoot symptoms to resolve in many cases 3 to 6 months after gastrocnemius recession.

In contrast, when surgically managing nonspastic gastrocsoleus equinus, this can be treated using the various techniques for tendoachilles lengthening procedures.[5] With regards to a tendoachilles lengthening procedure, meticulous care must be taken in the performance of the procedure, to avoid a devastating postoperative complication, calcaneal gait.[6]

Treatment for spastic soft tissue equinus differs from the nonspastic types. Most procedures to correct ankle equinus were originally described for the correction of spastic muscular equinus, as seen most notably in cerebral palsy. These procedures included neurectomies or proximal recessions, which were associated with high rates of complications and recurrence of the deformity. One effective approach described for the treatment of spastic equinus is the anterior advancement of the Achilles tendon, also known as Murphy tendoachilles advancement. This procedure shortens the lever arm of the Achilles tendon at the level of the ankle joint, decreasing its mechanical advantage and, thus, its power and resistance against dorsiflexion.[5]

Equinus of osseous origin can be addressed through a combination of osteotomies, arthrodeses, and concomitant soft tissue releases and tendon transfers. However, not only are these technically challenging, they are also associated with a high risk of complications, in particular, in the setting of associated infection or poor soft tissue envelope.[28] Additionally, complications relating to the neurovascular structures and skin have been reported with acute decrease in more severe deformities.[29] It would be both appropriate and beneficial to the surgeon to further delve into more advanced reconstructive options to avoid the aforementioned setbacks, which may be avoided through the use of external fixation.

EXTERNAL FIXATION FOR EQUINUS

Severe equinus contractures caused by trauma, burns, neurologic deficits, arthrogryposis, and osseous obstructions are usually not amenable to standard surgical treatments, including standard soft tissue releases, tendon transfers, and concomitant osseous procedures. In fact, performing acute correction of these severely contracted equinus deformities may have detrimental effects on the outcome of the surrounding soft tissue envelope and neurovascular structures.[30] In the case of contractures induced by burns or trauma, the resultant soft tissue defects are not responsive to posterior superficial muscle releases owing to their unstable poor skin and soft tissues.[31]

The benefits of using external fixation for the rectification of equinus are many. For one, gradual correction methods to correct simple or complex deformities decrease the operative exposure required when cutting bone. Additionally, the gentle gradual distraction that is possible with external fixation avoids acute stretch damage to the neurovascular structures and, thus, the magnitude of equinus correction required no longer becomes a barrier with progressive bone correction. It has been reported, however, that a tarsal tunnel release may be warranted when the correction angle of the equinus deformity required is more than 10°.[29,32] Bor and colleagues[30] mention a variety of skeletal conditions (eg, rickets) that are at risk for poor healing potential and require minimal disruption to their vascular-rich periosteal tissue. Minimal disruption of the soft tissue envelope is vital to the healing process and is, thus, possible through external fixation.

The concept of gradual correction of bone pioneered by Ilizarov stems from the idea that osseous structures respond to gradual mechanical distraction with new bone formation in a process called distraction osteogenesis. The simultaneous movement of the surrounding soft tissue during distraction is thus called distraction histogenesis.[33] The rate of distraction and correction was established by Herzenberg and Waanders to be a maximum of 1 mm per day at the fastest opening cortex or correcting segment, which was calculated using the rule of similar triangles. Experimental evidence suggests that low-load prolonged stretching is preferred compared with high-load brief intermittent collagen elongation.[30]

Most severe and noncorrectable equinus deformities can be addressed using either the closed or open Ilizarov treatment method. The closed method is reserved for children or adults with acceptable articular surfaces, joints, and bones. Open treatment uses osteotomies for correction if minimal articular surface and significant deformities are present, as seen, for example, in a neuropathic foot or in conditions that limit movement of the talus, that is, spurs.[23] There are 2 further variations of the Ilizarov method—the constrained or the unconstrained method.

The constrained method is used to correct the more rigid type of equinus deformity. This construct involves hinges, which are placed using the center of rotation of the ankle joint using Inman's axis, running through the distal aspect of the medial and lateral malleoli from anterior-medial-dorsal to posterior-lateral-plantar.[23,34] The construct starts with the tibial component, which has 2 tibial rings parallel to each other, attached to the leg via 2 or 3 crossing wires, and joined by 4 threaded rods. A horseshoe foot assembly connecting the hind, mid, and forefoot with a half ring placed at 90° over the metatarsals is subsequently placed angled at the same degree as the equinus deformity (**Fig. 2**), with 2 or 3 calcaneal wires with opposing olives placed under tension. Next, 2 or 3 wires with opposing olives are placed into the metatarsals, first through the fifth metatarsal base from lateral to medial, and second into the first metatarsal base from medial to lateral. Hinges are placed along the ankle joint axis. Precise placement and positioning of these hinges prevents anterior subluxation of the talus during correction. The distance between the rotation axis created by the hinges and the rods on the posterior foot and anterior foot constitute the leverage arms of the distraction and compression forces, respectively. The extent of distraction and traction forces on the respective threaded rods is directly proportional to the leverage arms.[23] The advantage of the constrained system is that the uniaxial hinge allows disconnection of the distraction rod with an active and passive range of motion of the joint being treated.[29] The negative to using this method is that the hinge system lined up on the center of the talar dome does not perfectly match the center of rotation of the ankle joint because the latter changes according to the ankle motion. This would thus require constant adjustment during the distraction process postoperatively to achieve ideal correction, which may be difficult from a practical standpoint and would be cumbersome.[32,34]

The unconstrained system uses a distraction technique to rotate around the center of the joint, essentially correcting itself around soft tissue hinges by using the natural axis of rotation of the joint. This method can be used for simple, unidirectional deformities and when bony deformities are not present.[23] The same tibial base of fixation with a simpler foot frame in this system, consisting of a half ring connecting posteriorly around the calcaneus, suspended off 2 or 3 threaded distraction rods locked by a nut distally and a hinge proximally. This posterior half ring is locked in with 2 crossing smooth or olive wires inserted through the heel, with distraction of the hindfoot being done in a posterior-inclined position. If distraction is performed in a purely axial direction parallel to the tibia, the talus tends to sublux anteriorly. The half ring attached anteriorly over the metatarsals with 2 crossing olive wires, one medially on the first

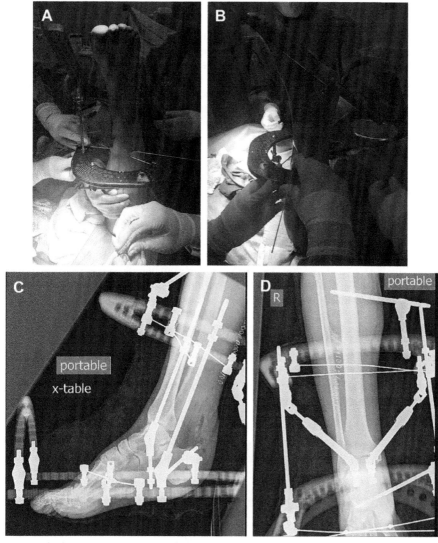

Fig. 2. (*A*) Placement of the footplate parallel to the equinus deformity. (*B*) Medial and lateral uniaxial hinge placement using the center of rotation of the ankle joint using In-man's axis. (*C*) Note on the radiograph hinges going through center of talar dome. (*D*) Universal hinged motors placed posteriorly perpendicular to the ankle joint axis to act as a push construct during gradual correction of the equinus deformity.

metatarsal and one laterally on the fifth metatarsal, connects to the tibial ring with threaded compression rods. Metatarsal dorsiflexion requires hinges distally on the metatarsal ring and a rotating post proximally at the tibial ring to allow the metatarsal pin to translate anteriorly as the deformity is corrected. Additionally, the ankle joint must be distracted 2 to 5 mm compared with preoperative radiographs to limit cartilage compression and midfoot rockerbottom deformity. The advantage of the unconstrained system is that it is simpler to apply and is more forgiving than the constrained method, because the correction is done around the natural axes of rotation of the joints and soft tissue hinges, and not through a precisely placed pair of hinges along the defined anatomic axis of the joint.[23,29,30]

DiDomenico and associates[35] report an alternative technique for transosseous calcaneal pinning where oblique half pins, instead of 2 crossing wires, are placed from the posterior calcaneus toward the medial and lateral column, allowing for increased control of the calcaneus. The pins can subsequently be inserted into the midfoot once the calcaneus has been manipulated into place, allowing for stabilization and correction of the hindfoot to the midfoot as a single construct. This orientation of pin insertion allows for pins to stay away from vital neurovascular structures and for better visualization during placement.[35]

THESE AUTHORS' METHOD USING EXTERNAL FIXATION FOR THE TREATMENT OF EQUINUS: GRADUAL
Securing the Tibial Block

A hip bump is placed under the hip of the ipsilateral limb to have the knee straight vertically in the transverse plane and a bump is placed under the knee above the level of the tibial block. A tibial block made up of 2 parallel rings is applied at the distal one-third of the tibia. Each tibial ring is secured with a 5-mm half-pin placed into the medial face of the tibia with additional crossing 1.8 mm smooth wires in standard fashion tensioned to 130 kg. When using a short footplate or a five-eighth's ring, the wires are tensioned at a lower magnitude of approximately 90 kg to disallow deforming forces at the open segment. Medial face half pins should be divergent from the tibial rings at 30° to 45° in all cardinal planes. The authors prefer not to violate the anterior tibial crest or the lateral face of the tibia to avoid stress risers and neurovascular damage, respectively. Placement of half pins should be checked under fluoroscopy to ensure proper placement and position with 2 to 3 threads penetrating the opposing tibial cortex (**Fig. 3**).

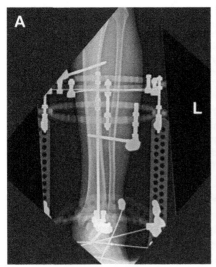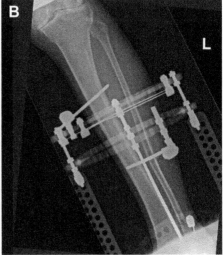

Fig. 3. Placement of threaded half pins in the medial face of the tibia divergent from the tibial ring in all cardinal planes, promoting a more stabilized tibial block construct. (*A*) Anterior posterior tibia fibula view of buttress frame. (*B*) Oblique tibia fibula view of buttress frame.

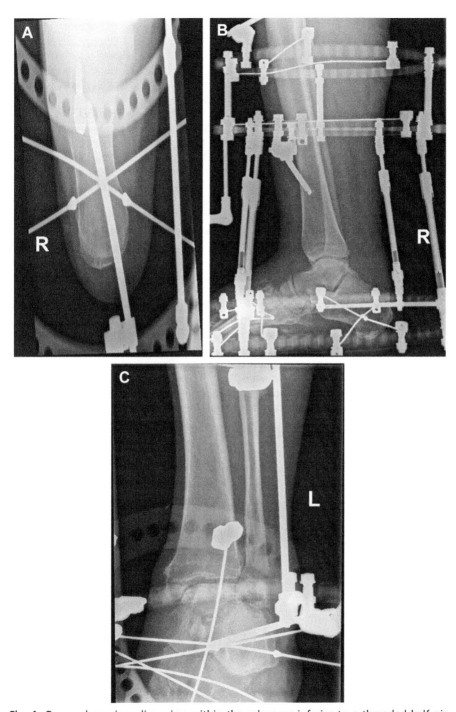

Fig. 4. Opposed crossing olive wires within the calcaneus inferior to a threaded half pin from posterior to anterior. This configuration protects the integrity of the half pin while increasing the rigidity of the hindfoot construct. (*A*) Calcaneal axial view of apical half pin. (*B*) Lateral ankle view of crossing olive wire, apical half pin, placed perpendicular to the calcaneal cuboid joint. (*C*) Medial oblique view of the configuration.

Securing the Footplate

The footplate is initially secured using a posteromedial to anterolateral directed half pin within the calcaneus perpendicular to the calcaneocuboid joint and parallel to the weightbearing surface. Two crossed opposing olive wires are placed medially and laterally inferior to the half pin in the calcaneal tuberosity at approximately 45° to 60° from each other and are tensioned to 90 kg in a closed footplate construct. This configuration of the opposed crossed olive wires protects the integrity of the half pin within the calcaneus, while simultaneously increasing the rigidity of the construct (**Fig. 4**). A lateral 1.8-mm metatarsal olive wire is placed starting at the proximal fifth metatarsal aiming dorsal distal in an attempt to intersect the fifth , fourth, and second metatarsals. A second medial olive wire is inserted from the proximal first metatarsal and aimed slightly anterior and plantar to engage the first, third, and fourth metatarsals. Wire placement is checked under fluoroscopy in the anteroposterior and lateral views to confirm placement (**Fig. 5**). Wires can also be placed into the midfoot, but wire insertion into the metatarsals maximizes the lever arm and the mechanical advantage.

Gradual Correction with Ankle Axis Hinges

Once the tibial block and footplate are attached, an ankle axis wire, matching Inman's axis, is inserted from anterior-medial-dorsal to posterior-lateral-plantar just distal to the malleoli into the talus, and threaded rods are used to attach the Ilizarov hinges to the external fixator. Once the hinges have been connected to the external fixator, the ankle axis wire is removed. Universally hinged motors are then placed perpendicularly to the ankle axis, posteriorly, and/or anteriorly. These motors will be the generators for the force correcting the equinus (**Fig. 2D**). The universal hinges on the motors permit the ankle to undergo dorsiflexion/plantarflexion, eversion/supination, and abduction/adduction as the equinus deformity is corrected.

Gradual Correction with the Hexapod System

Equinus correction can also be achieved with a hexapod construct. Using this configuration, the surgeon can forego the use of an ankle axis wire and use a

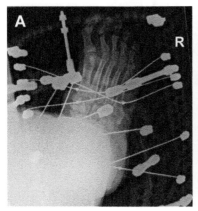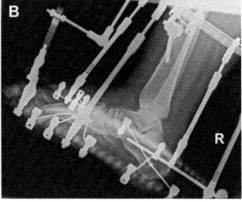

Fig. 5. Opposed crossing olive wires in the forefoot, one medially from the base of the first metatarsal and one laterally from the base of the fifth metatarsal. (*A*) Oblique Foot Xray displaying bent and tensioned metatarsal wires. (*B*) Lateral view of ankle displaying the bent wire technique of the midtarsus with equinus correction on standard foot plate.

computer-aided correction plan. Mounting the tibial block to the footplate occurs using multidirectional motors. These motors are mounted between the tibial block and the footplate (**Fig. 6**).

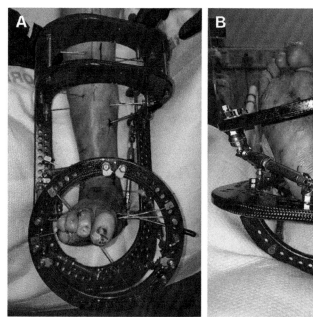
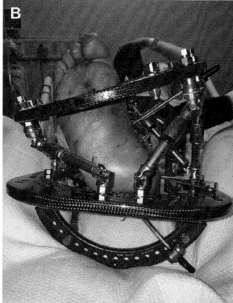
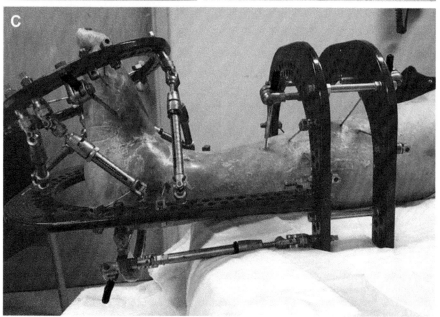

Fig. 6. Gradual correction of midfoot Charcot breakdown with equinus in the rearfoot and a varus rotation in the forefoot using a hexapod construct. (*A*) Anterior posterior view of hexapod gradual buttress frame configuration. (*B*) Plantar view displaying offset calcaneal half pin. (*C*) Lateral view of Hexapod Gradual buttress frame configuration.

THESE AUTHORS' METHOD USING EXTERNAL FIXATION FOR THE TREATMENT OF EQUINUS: ACUTE

The authors' preference when correcting equinus acutely as part of a more complex deformity is through the use of a static external fixator. This static frame can be in either a buttress configuration or a standard configuration. The author attaches the frame using the techniques previously outlined. A Hoke triple hemisection of the Achilles tendon is performed. A 5- or 6-mm half pin is placed from a posterior, slightly medial approach, targeted toward a perpendicular bisector of the calcaneo-cuboid joint, inferior to the subtalar joint. Care is taken not to violate the calcaneo-cuboid and subtalar joints. This calcaneal half pin can now be used as a joystick to correct the equinus deformity acutely (**Fig. 7**). Intraoperative measurements are taken to determine if correction was achieved. The anatomic tibial bisector should now pass through the lateral process of the talus, and the calcaneal inclination and tibiotalar angle should be corrected. If there is residual talar declination, a posterior capsular release is performed through a 5-cm incision made lateral to the Achilles tendon. Dissection is performed to the level of the deep fascia. A Cobb elevator is used to dissect the adhered ankle capsule that is impeding the talar component of the equinus. Once adequate correction is achieved using the joystick half-pin method, the half pin is subsequently secured to the posterior footplate. In the buttress frame configuration, the pin is secured to a 3/8 ring attached perpendicularly to the posterior aspect of the long footplate at the level of the calcaneus (**Fig. 8**).

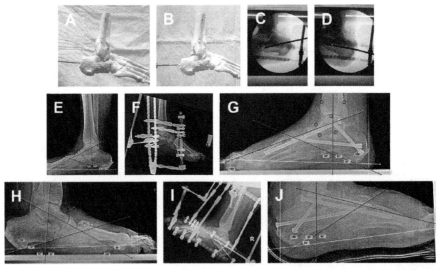

Fig. 7. Saw bone schematic with a threaded half pin in the posterior calcaneus placed orthogonal to the long axis of the bone (A) in an uncorrected position and (B) in a corrected position. (C) Intraoperative fluoroscopy demonstrating the use of a threaded half pin to "joystick" the calcaneus out of a plantarflex position (D) to a more dorsiflexed, corrected position. (E, H) Preoperative radiographs. (F, I) Intraoperative radiographs. (G, J) Postoperative radiographs with definitive percutaneous placed internal fixation to hold the correction after frame removal in 2 patients—increased calcaneal inclination and decreased talar declination angle in both.

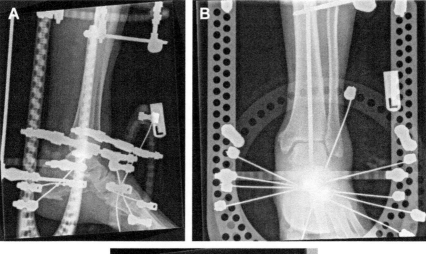

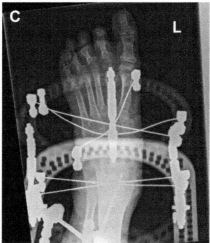

Fig. 8. Buttress frame configuration with pin secured to a 3/8 ring attached perpendicularly to the posterior aspect of the long footplate at the level of the calcaneus. (*A*) Lateral view of Acute Buttress configuration with perpendicular forefoot wire placement. (*B*) Anterior Posterior view of Buttress Frame displaying Perpendicular forefoot wire placement. (*C*) Anterior posterior view.

SUMMARY

Equinus is considered to be one of the most destructive forces and has been directly correlated with a large number of pathologies of the foot and ankle. Although there has been a recent push for being more cognizant of it, a high rate of underdiagnosis and misdiagnosis of the deformity remains. There are a variety of treatment options, ranging from conservative therapy to standard surgical means, which include soft tissue releases, osteotomies, and tendon transfers to name a few that are helpful to patients with more of a mild to moderate type of equinus deformity.

The foot and ankle surgeon, however, has to be prepared to face and address more severely contracted types of equinus deformity that are not acquiescent to treatment via these options. Trauma, severe burn contractures, neuromuscular disease, polio-myelitis, Charcot neuroarthropathy, neglected or relapsed clubfoot, and osseous obstruction at the tibiotalar joint are some of the more common etiologies of the severe type of nonreducible equinus that fail treatment with conventional methods. Further-more, owing to the severity of the deformity and the poor soft tissue construct often seen with these diseases, addressing their related equinus deformity through the sole use of the standard surgical approaches may require extensive wedge bone re-sections, which would not only be difficult, but could also harm the surrounding soft tissue and leave the patient with a shortened foot.[36] This is where the role of external fixation in the treatment of equinus comes in, for which a variety of techniques have been reported in the past.

Deformities, such as equinocavovarus, which has equinus as one of its compo-nents, must be corrected in multiple planes. Although this correction is possible through the use of conventional frames with universal hinges, the introduction of a hexapod external fixator has made the reconstruction of these pathologies more effi-cient with reproducible outcomes. Nomura and colleagues[37] reports the use of a Tay-lor spatial frame for the correction of a poliomyelitic equinocavovarus foot. These frame types allow for simultaneous correction of multifaceted deformities that are computer based, making things more convenient for the surgeon.[38]

Some of the complications with the use of external fixation for treatment of equinus include pin site infections, noncompliance, subluxation of joints during the correction process, and claw toe deformity to name a few. There have been reports of flexor tendon releases, or fixation of K-wires across digital joints to prevent claw toe forma-tion during the distraction process.[29,36,39] Yet, one of the most common complications is the recurrence of the deformity after the removal of the external fixator. Long-term bracing (6 to 12 months duration) and physical therapy have shown to help maintain soft tissue correction.[29] However, Melvin and Dahners[34] have reported, based on their study, that factors such as etiology or duration of the contracture, rather than duration of the corrective force, affected whether the deformity recurs in the long term. They found that an etiology of burn contracture, a long duration of contracture, and a large contracture before surgery correlated with an inability to maintain correction.

All in all, the goal of this article was to provide an overview of the topic of equinus, which included the biomechanics, classification, etiologies, clinical identification, and standard treatment of it. However, more than anything else, it also served to review previous reported indications and techniques, as well as the author's own techniques for the use of external fixation when managing severe, nonreducible equinus deformity that are not treatable through conventional means.

REFERENCES

1. Clifford C. Understanding the biomechanics of equinus. Podiatry Today 2014; 27(9):1–11.
2. Digiovanni CW, Kuo R, Tejwani N, et al. Isolated gastrocnemius tightness. J Bone Joint Surg Am 2002;84-A(6):962–70.
3. Johnson CH, Christensen JC. Biomechanics of the first ray part V: the effect of equinus deformity, a 3-dimensional kinematic study on a cadaver model. J Foot Ankle Surg 2005;44(1):114–20.
4. Barrett SL. Understanding and managing equinus deformities. Podiatry Today 2011;24(5):58–66.
5. Downey MS. Current surgical procedures for lengthening of the triceps surae and its components. In: McGlamry ED, editor. Reconstructive surgery of the foot and

leg – update '88. Tucker (GA): Podiatry Institute Publishing Company; 1988. p. 97–104.

6. DeHeer PA. Equinus and lengthening techniques. Clin Podiatr Med Surg 2017; 34:207–27.

7. Wren TA, Do KP, Kay RM. Gastrocnemius and soleus lengths in cerebral palsy equinus gait—differences between children with and without static contracture and effects of gastrocnemius recession. J Biomech 2004;37(9):1321–7.

8. Perry J. Gait analysis: normal and pathological function (2nd edition), Chapter 11, ankle and foot gait deviations. Second edition. Thorofare (NJ): Slack Inc; 2010.

9. Yoon KS, Park SD. The effects of ankle mobilization and active stretching on the difference of weight-bearing distribution, low back pain and flexibility in pronated-foots subjects. J Exerc Rehabil 2013;9(2):292–7.

10. Gourdine-Shaw MC, Lamm BM, Herzenberg JE, et al. Equinus deformity in the pediatric patient: causes, evaluation, and management. Clin Podiatr Med Surg 2010;27:25–42.

11. Charles J, Scutter SD, Buckley J. Static ankle joint equinus toward a standard definition and diagnosis. J Am Podiatr Med Assoc 2010;100(3):195–203.

12. Barouk P, Barouk LS. Clinical diagnosis of gastrocnemius tightness. Foot Ankle Clin N Am 2014;19:659–67.

13. Downey MS, Schwartz JM. Ankle equinus. In: Southerland JT, Boberg JS, Downey MS, et al, editors. McGlamry's comprehensive textbook of foot and ankle surgery. 4th edition. New York: Lippincott William & Wilkins; 2013. p. 541–85.

14. Grimston SK, Nigg BM, Hanley DA. Differences in ankle joint complex range of motion as a function of age. Foot Ankle 1993;14:215–22.

15. Muellenbach EA, Diehl CJ, Teachey MK, et al. Interactions of the advanced glycation end product inhibitor pyridoxamine and the antioxidant α-lipoic acid on insulin resistance in the obese Zucker rat. Metabolism 2008;57:1465–72.

16. Ulrich P, Cerami A. Protein glycation, diabetes, and aging. Recent Prog Horm Res 2001;56:1–21.

17. Grant WP, Sullivan R, Sonenshine DE, et al. Electron microscopic investigation of the effects of diabetes mellitus on the Achilles tendon. J Foot Ankle Surg 1997;36: 272–8.

18. Giacomozzi C, D'Amrogi E, Uccioli L, et al. Does the thickening of Achilles tendon and plantar fascia contribute to the alteration of diabetic foot loading? Clin Biomech 2005;20:532–9.

19. DiGiovanni CW, Holt S, Czerniecki JM, et al. Can the presence of equinus contracture be established by physical exam alone? J Rehabil Res Dev 2001; 38(3):335–40.

20. Woods C, Hawkins RD, Maltby S, et al. The football association medical research programme: an audit of injuries in professional football: analysis of hamstring injuries. Br J Sports Med 2004;38:36–41.

21. Jaberzadeh S, Scutter S, Nazeran H. Mechanosensitivity of the median nerve and mechanically produced motor responses during upper limb neurodynamic test 1. Physiotherapy 2005;91:94.

22. Gatt A, De Giorgio S, Chockalingam N, et al. A pilot investigation into the relationship between static diagnosis of ankle equinus and dynamic ankle and foot dorsiflexion during stance phase of gait: time to revisit theory? Foot (Edinb) 2017;30: 47–52.

23. Kirienko A, Villa A, Calhoun JH. The equinus foot. In: Kirienko A, Villa A, Calhoun JH, editors. Ilizarov technique for complex foot and ankle deformities. 1st edition. New York: Marcel Dekker, Inc; 2004. p. 25–57.

24. Elomrani N, Kasis A, Saleh M. A radiographic technique for the assessment of ankle and midfoot equinus. Foot Ankle Int 2005;26(3):251–5.
25. Grady JF, Saxena A. Effects of stretching the gastrocnemius muscle. J Foot Surg 1991;30(5):465–9.
26. Evans A. Podiatric medical applications of posterior night stretch splinting. J Am Podiatr Med Assoc 2001;91(7):356–60.
27. DiGiovanni CW, Langer P. The role of isolated gastrocnemius and combined Achilles contractures in the flatfoot. Foot Ankle Clin 2007;12(2):363–78, viii.
28. Jeong BO, Kim TY, Song WJ. Use of Ilizarov external fixation without soft tissue release to correct severe, rigid equinus deformity. J Foot Ankle Surg 2015;54:821–5.
29. Mendicino RW, Murphy LJ, Maskill MP, et al. Application of a constrained external fixator frame for treatment of a fixed equinus contracture. J Foot Ankle Surg 2008; 47(5):468–75.
30. Bor N, Rubin G, Rozen N. Ilizarov method for gradual deformity correction. Oper Tech Orthop 2011;21:104–12.
31. Hahn SB, Park HJ, Park HW, et al. Treatment of severe equinus deformity associated with extensive scarring of the leg. Clin Orthop Relat Res 2001;393:250–7.
32. Tsuchiya H, Sakurakichi K, Uehara K, et al. Gradual closed correction of equinus contracture using the Ilizarov apparatus. J Orthop Sci 2003;8:802–6.
33. Tetsworth K, Paley D. Basic science of distraction histogenesis. Curr Opin Orthop 1995;6:61–8.
34. Melvin JS, Dahners LE. A technique for correction of equinus contracture using a wire fixator and elastic tension. J Orthop Trauma 2006;20:138–42.
35. DiDomenico LA, Giagnacova A, Cross DJ, et al. An alternative technique for transosseous calcaneal pinning in external fixation. J Foot Ankle Surg 2012; 51(4):528–30.
36. Kocaoglu M, Eralp L, Atalar AC, et al. Correction of complex foot deformities using the Ilizarov external fixator. J Foot Ankle Surg 2002;41(1):30–9.
37. Nomura I, Watanabe K, Matsubara H, et al. Correction of a severe poliomyelitic equinocavovarus foot using an adjustable external fixation frame. J Foot Ankle Surg 2014;53:235–8.
38. Wukich DK, Dial D. Equinovarus deformity correction with the Taylor spatial frame. Oper Tech Orthop 2006;16:18–22.
39. Lamm B, Paley D, Testani M, et al. Tarsal tunnel decompression in leg lengthening and deformity correction of the foot and ankle. J Foot Ankle Surg 2007; 463:201–6.

Lengthen, Alignment, and Beam Technique for Midfoot Charcot Neuroarthropathy

Guido A. LaPorta, DPM, MS[a,b,*], Alison D'Andelet, DPM, MHA[a]

KEYWORDS

- Charcot neuroarthropathy • Superconstructs • LAB technique • Osteomyelitis
- Hexapod • External fixation

KEY POINTS

- Charcot neuroarthropathy is a devastating and disabling pathology in the foot and ankle, particularly when affecting the midfoot.
- When the midfoot is affected, there is frequently development of a rocker-bottom deformity, owing to progressive subluxation and dislocation, primarily of the lateral column.
- Patients with midfoot Charcot neuroarthropathy, particularly those with current or prior ulceration, are at high risk for infection, amputation, and even mortality if the deformity is not addressed.

INTRODUCTION

Charcot neuroarthropathy is a devastating and disabling pathology in the foot and ankle, particularly when affecting the midfoot. Of the 30.3 million people in the United States currently diagnosed with diabetes, approximately 0.5% will develop Charcot neuroarthropathy at some point in their lives.[1,2] Sanders and Frykberg, as well as Brodsky and Rouse, classified the anatomic patterns of involvement in Charcot neuroarthropathy, and determined that the tarsometatarsal joint and/or midtarsal joints are most commonly involved.[3,4] The prevalence of the deformity at this anatomic location prompted Schon and Sammarco to each further classify midfoot Charcot in 1998.[5] When the midfoot is affected, there is frequently development of a "rocker-bottom" deformity, owing to progressive subluxation and dislocation, primarily of the lateral column. Additionally, the presence of an equinus deformity secondary to motor and sensory neuropathy and subsequent motor imbalance can increase forces in and on the midfoot, further

Disclosure: The authors have nothing to disclose.
[a] Podiatric Medical Education, Our Lady of Lourdes Memorial Hospital, 169 Riverside Dr, Binghamton, NY 13905, USA; [b] Podiatric Medical Education, Geisinger-Community Medical Center, 1800 Mulberry St, Scranton, PA 18510, USA
* Corresponding author. Podiatric Medical Education, Geisinger-Community Medical Center, 1800 Mulberry St, Scranton, PA 18510.
E-mail address: glaporta@msn.com

Clin Podiatr Med Surg 35 (2018) 497–507
https://doi.org/10.1016/j.cpm.2018.05.008
0891-8422/18/© 2018 Elsevier Inc. All rights reserved.

podiatric.theclinics.com

contributing to collapse.[6] The Achilles tendon is also abnormal in diabetic patients secondary to glycation of the collagen fibers, causing increased stiffness and higher peak plantar pressures.[7] The abnormal plantar pedal pressure and shearing forces resulting from the midfoot deformity increases the risk of ulceration, osteomyelitis, and possible amputation.[8] A study by Sohn and colleagues[9] found that diabetic patients with Charcot neuroarthropathy alone had a risk of amputation 7 times greater than patients with neuropathic foot ulcerations and a risk of amputation 12 times greater if they had an ulcer secondary to the Charcot deformity. Thus, patients with midfoot Charcot neuroarthropathy, particularly those with current or prior ulceration, are at high risk for infection, amputation, and even mortality if the deformity is not addressed.

The goals in treating Charcot neuroarthropathy are to create a stable and plantigrade foot, with no open wounds or infection, that can be placed in a shoe or brace. However, these goals are not often achievable with conservative treatment in patients with midfoot pathology because of the propensity of the plantar tissue to break down, as well as the difficulty in finding shoe gear to accommodate the plantar prominence of the rocker-bottom deformity.[10,11] In these cases, surgical reconstruction of the foot is often required to restore function and decrease the risk of amputation secondary to ulceration and infection. There are many procedures that can be considered in treating midfoot deformities, ranging from plantar exostectomy and tendo-Achilles lengthening to realignment of advanced deformity with internal and/or external fixation. There is no available evidence in the literature that suggests the superiority of any proposed surgical intervention or fixation technique. In this article, we describe the approach we use in correcting midfoot Charcot deformities.

SURGICAL TECHNIQUE

Surgical correction of midfoot Charcot arthropathy is achieved via the 2-step lengthen, alignment, and beam (LAB) technique. The first step of the LAB technique involves acute correction of the equinus deformity and gradual correction of the deformity using computer-assisted hexapod external fixation. An Achilles tendon lengthening is performed first, to allow the rearfoot to be placed in a neutral position. This step is necessary to achieve anatomic correction of the midfoot. We generally prefer to perform an open tendo-Achilles lengthening. A percutaneous lengthening is indicated if there is a significant equinus deformity, owing to the ability to achieve a greater amount of lengthening.[12] The tendo-Achilles lengthening is performed via a medial incision to decrease the risk of complications to the neurovascular structures along the lateral aspect of the gastrocnemius aponeurosis.

Gradual correction and alignment is preferred, because it allows for the correction of significant multiplanar deformities while maintaining foot length and bone mass and reducing risk of neurovascular compromise. This approach can be used in either an acute or coalesced deformity; however, an osteotomy is required if the deformity is coalesced to allow for anatomic reduction of the bony segments. Ideally, the osteotomy should be placed at the apex of the deformity to allow for maximal correction. The type of osteotomy required depends on the deformity present and should be determined using preoperative radiographs. In actuality, the osteotomy can only be performed within the confines of the lesser tarsus, regardless of whether or not it corresponds with the deformity apex. It is our preference to perform open osteotomies in patients with a coalesced deformity, although percutaneous osteotomies can also be performed using a Gigli saw. Osteotomies are not typically required in cases where there is bony dissolution or nonunion of midfoot fractures, because the foot remains unstable and able to be manipulated. The hexapod external fixator is then applied to gradually distract (lengthen) and realign the bony segments. The most commonly used construct is a 6 × 6 butt frame, which allows for gradual correction of the forefoot on a fixed hindfoot. The technique used is referred to as a rings-first, distal reference, 180° offset 6 × 6 Hexapod (**Fig. 1**). It may be necessary to fuse the subtalar joint to produce a stabile hindfoot. Once the frame is in place, orthogonal radiographs are obtained in the operating room or immediately postoperatively. These radiographs provide information required for the software program, which in turn provides a prescription with daily strut adjustments. As the struts are adjusted, the midfoot deformity is reduced into a corrected position over a 17- to 24-day period (**Fig. 2**). Pin sites are cleaned on a weekly basis with sterile saline. Once the program is complete, the patient returns to the operating room for the second stage of the process.

The second step of the LAB technique involves removal of the external fixator and minimally invasive beaming of the medial and lateral columns. Joint preparation occurs either via 1- to 2-cm incisions at each joint location or a 10-cm incision along each column. Joint surfaces are then resected via rongeur, sagittal saw, or trephine technique, and a flexible drill bit is used to pierce the subchondral bone (**Fig. 3**). In some cases, the use of a trephine is preferred to excise the diseased joint articulations and the subsequent deficit can be packed with bone matrix or an allograft dowel (**Fig. 4**). Platelet-rich plasma or bone marrow aspirate are also frequently used when preparing the joints for beaming. When beaming the medial column, the first metatarsophalangeal joint is opened through a dorsal incision and the metatarsal head is released from its surrounding soft tissue attachments. As the guidewire from the 7.0/8.0-mm cannulated screw set is inserted through the distal aspect of the metatarsal head and driven into the body of the talus, it can also be used as a joystick to ensure the appropriate alignment is achieved, restoring the normal relationship between the talus and first metatarsal. The position can then be confirmed on fluoroscopy, with the guidewire passing through the medullary canal of the first metatarsal and through the head and neck of the talus, without violating the ankle or subtalar joints. A cannulated drill is used only on the metatarsal head, and then a 7.0/8.0-mm screw is inserted and buried into the metatarsal head. The lateral column beaming is performed in a similar fashion, with a dorsal incision placed over the fourth metatarsal phalangeal joint. The fourth metatarsal is frequently chosen because it is

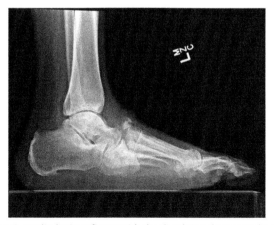

Fig. 1. The construct is applied "rings first," with the distal ring designated as the reference ring and the master tab rotated 180° so that it is located on the plantar aspect of the foot. (*From* Rubin Institute for Advanced Orthopedics, Sinai Hospital of Baltimore, 2018; with permission.)

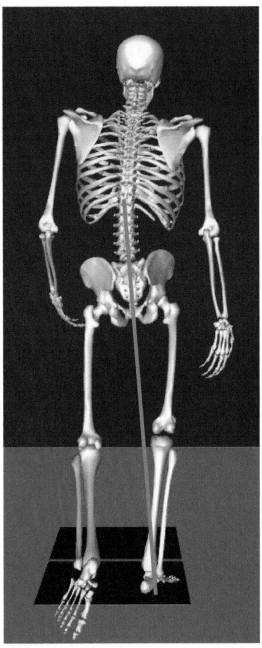

Fig. 2. Correction and final alignment typically takes 17 to 24 days. (*From* Rubin Institute for Advanced Orthopedics, Sinai Hospital of Baltimore, 2018; with permission.)

more in line with the cuboid and calcaneus. Once the metatarsal head is released from the soft tissue attachments, the guidewire is placed through the distal metatarsal head and driven through the cuboid into the lateral calcaneus. Again, a cannulated drill is used only on the metatarsal head, and a 5.0- to 7.0-mm screw is inserted and buried. Frequently, the diameter of the fourth metatarsal is too small to pass a 5.0- to 7.0-mm

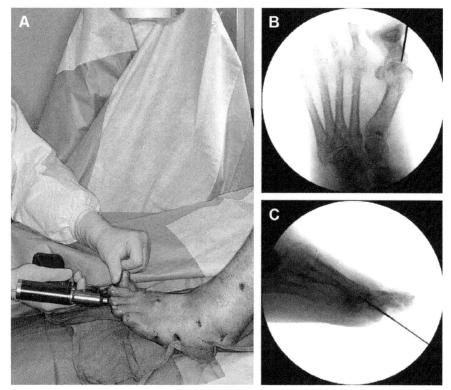

Fig. 3. A flexible 2.7-mm drill is used to fenestrate joint surfaces. (*A*) Clinical photograph (*B*) AP view of the flexible drill under fluoroscopy (*C*) Lateral view of the flexible drill under fluoroscopy. (*From* Rubin Institute for Advanced Orthopedics, Sinai Hospital of Baltimore, 2018; with permission.)

beam and the fixation must start at the base of the metatarsal (**Fig. 5**). Adequate position and compression is confirmed with fluoroscopy. Additional intramedullary fixation can be placed as needed through the second or third metatarsal for increased stability. The patient is then placed into a short leg cast with the foot at 90° and remains nonweightbearing for approximately 10 to 12 weeks. Protected weightbearing is then allowed based on radiographic appearance.

This technique can also be modified for cases where there is osteomyelitis present at the midfoot secondary to current or prior ulceration. In these cases, during the preliminary procedure, all infected bone is resected and antibiotic beads or spacers are placed in the void. The antibiotic beads can dissolve or be removed surgically, depending on surgeon preference of drug delivery materials. A hexapod external fixator can be applied at this time to provide stabilization. Any remaining necrotic soft tissue or bone can also be removed during the first stage. Additionally, if there is concern about bone loss secondary to resection of infected bone, an antibiotic-infused allograft can be used during the second stage of the LAB technique to restore length and provide continued local antibiotic delivery.

DISCUSSION

Charcot neuroarthropathy of the midfoot can have a significant effect on patients' ability to function and their quality of life. There are multiple ways to address midfoot

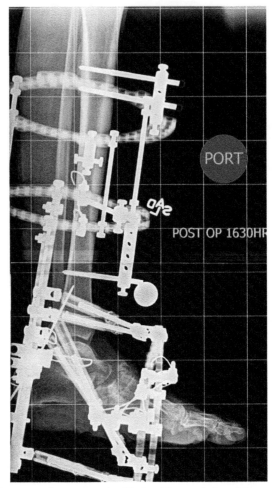

Fig. 4. Joint surfaces may be prepared with trephine and dowel bone graft to facilitate fusion. (*From* Rubin Institute for Advanced Orthopedics, Sinai Hospital of Baltimore, 2018; with permission.)

Charcot deformities, but there is no gold standard in treating midfoot Charcot owing to the variety in presentations secondary to acuity, stability, location, and presence of ulceration and/or infection. These various components of the pathology require careful consideration by the surgeon with regard to how best to manage each patient's particular deformity. The goal, however, remains the same regardless of these details—to restore a stable, plantigrade foot, with no ulcerations, which can be placed in a brace or shoe. The 2-step LAB technique described in this article is not presented as a superior method of treating midfoot Charcot, but rather an alternative treatment option that can be considered (**Fig. 6**).

The greatest benefit of the LAB technique is the melding of the use of internal and external fixation. The use of a hexapod during the first stage provides multiple advantages. The external fixator provides rigid stability to the osseous components and offloading of the soft tissues, allowing for management of edema and preexisting soft

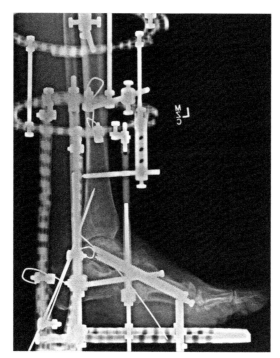

Fig. 5. The wire is introduced through the first metatarsal head and directed toward the talar head facilitated by fluoroscopic imaging. The wire is placed on a trajectory that allows placement in the talar head and neck. Frequently, the diameter of the fourth metatarsal is too small to pass a 5.0- to 7.0-mm beam and the fixation must start at the base of the metatarsal. (*From* Rubin Institute for Advanced Orthopedics, Sinai Hospital of Baltimore, 2018; with permission.)

tissue defects.[13] The hexapod-assisted gradual correction achieved during the first stage of the procedure allows for more accurate anatomic alignment than could ever be achieved with manual reduction in an acute correction, while also providing stability.[14] The hexapod external fixation system has been shown to have a

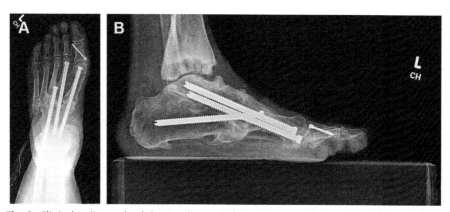

Fig. 6. Clinical radiographs. (*A*) AP radiograph following second step of the LAB technique. (*B*) Lateral radiograph following second step of the LAB technique. (*From* Rubin Institute for Advanced Orthopedics, Sinai Hospital of Baltimore, 2018; with permission.)

mechanical accuracy within 0.7° and 2 mm and mathematical accuracy of 1/1,000,000 inches in correction of 6-axis deformity.[15] Thus, the LAB technique is best used for patients who have large angular deformities in multiple planes, or subluxation through the midfoot with no significant bony defects or fractures, because this technique allows for the precise realignment of joints without loss of foot length or bone mass. The gradual correction also protects the soft tissue and neurovascular structures, which are often contracted in long-standing deformities and can be compromised in acute corrections, and allows for minimal incisions and dissection in tissues with poor healing potential.[13,16] The external fixator also provides a way for the surgeon to address cases where there is osteomyelitis present, allowing for resection of infected bone, local antibiotic delivery, and subsequent stabilization or correction of deformity with placement of internal fixation once the infection is resolved.[13,17]

There are inherent challenges in using standard internal fixation techniques to address Charcot neuroarthropathy, namely because of the significant degree of deformity and bony resorption that occur as part of the pathology.[18,19] In addition to the poor bone quality in these patients, neuropathy, vascular disease, and poor nutrition also can delay healing and contribute to complications when performing reconstructions.[18] These barriers in treating midfoot Charcot led to the concept of "superconstructs," which are surgical techniques used in these cases to improve stability and decrease fixation failure. Superconstructs have 4 defining features: fusion beyond the zone of injury to include normal joints, bony resection to allow for shortening of the extremity and adequate deformity reduction without excessive soft tissue tension, use of the strongest possible device tolerated by the soft tissue, and application of the fixation device in a position that maximizes its mechanical function. Axial screw placement, or intramedullary beaming, is one of these superconstructs, along with plantar plating and locking plates.[18]

Intramedullary beaming, the second stage of the LAB technique, has many advantages compared with plate fixation. Intramedullary beaming allows for the internal fixation device to accept tension on both the dorsal and plantar surfaces, and increases contact area between the bone and fixation, providing increased stability.[19,20] A cadaveric study performed by Pope and colleagues[21] found no difference between intramedullary beaming and plantar plating with regard to stiffness, hardware failure, or loads to failure. Thus, the stability benefits of the plantar plate can be achieved with intramedullary beaming without the need for the extensive dissection and periosteal stripping that the placement of a plantar plate requires.[19,20] The trabecular bone quality present in patients with Charcot neuroarthropathy has been found to be weaker and less organized than normal trabecular bone, which can increase failure risk with hardware, such as plates or oblique screws owing to loss of bone purchase.[22] The intramedullary position of the screw makes it more inherently stable, even in weaker bone, and also eliminates stress risers in the cortical bone of the metatarsals that can occur with plates or oblique screws.[18] Intramedullary beaming assists in reduction of the deformity, particularly the medial column sag in the sagittal plane, and resists deforming forces within the sagittal and transverse planes.[19] The screws are also placed via small incisions and are completely intraosseous, allowing the bone and soft tissue to act as a biologic barrier to protect the hardware in cases of wound dehiscence.[19,23] A study by Cullen and colleagues[24] evaluated use of the midfoot intramedullary nail and experienced an incident in one of their cases in which a deep abscess formed along the lateral incision site, but they were able to maintain the implanted hardware through achievement of bony union because it was not compromised by the soft tissue infection as a plate might have been.

Although intramedullary beaming has proven to be a viable option for treatment of midfoot Charcot in the literature, there remains some debate regarding the specifics of the screw. The principles of intramedullary nailing in long bones should be applied in this situation as well with regard to choosing an appropriate size screw. The screw ideally will cross a healthy joint proximal and distal to the affected bones, allowing for a bridging of the area to achieve increased stability. Likewise, the screw should fill the intramedullary canal without compromising the cortical bone, increasing the contact area between the fixation and bone. This generally means that the screw size chosen should be the longest and largest screw able to cross the entire medial or lateral column.[18,20] Typically, this means the screw ranges in size from 6.5 to 8.0 mm, depending on the patient.

The material properties of the screws used for midfoot beaming have also been discussed in the literature. It is our preference to use a cannulated screw, because it allows for fluoroscopic visualization throughout the placement of the guidewire and screw to ensure appropriate position and alignment. A solid screw, however, must be inserted after the removal of a guidewire, which can make placement more technically difficult. The benefit of the solid screw is its increased strength relative to a cannulated screw. A study by Sammarco and colleagues[25] experienced breakage of 36.4% of their 6.5-mm cannulated screws, whereas studies by Wiewiorski and colleagues[26] and Cullen and colleagues[24] found no breakage of their 6.5-mm solid screws. There is also comparison of titanium and stainless steel screws. Stainless steel fixation has been shown to have greater tensile strength, greater resistance to load-bearing stress, and longer fatigue failure rate over time when compared with titanium. However, titanium does have better biocompatibility, improved bone adherence, and absence of allergic response, which may outweigh the limitation of durability in some patients.[19]

The LAB technique is also an excellent approach to managing concurrent midfoot Charcot neuroarthropathy and osteomyelitis. Osteomyelitis is an additional complicating factor; the abnormal plantar pedal pressure and shearing forces resulting from the midfoot deformity increases the risk of ulceration and osteomyelitis.[8] It is our practice that patients suspected of having osteomyelitis and Charcot undergo bone scintigraphy with an initial leukocyte scan, followed by a marrow scan (sulfur colloid) if the leukocyte scan is positive. If there is increased uptake of labeled leukocytes to a particular site without a corresponding uptake of sulfur colloid at the same site, osteomyelitis is present. If there is concordance in the uptake of leukocyte and marrow imaging, it can be assumed that Charcot neuroarthropathy is present without concurrent infection.[27,28] This combined scintigraphy improves the diagnostic accuracy within the diabetic foot, with a sensitivity of 92% and specificity of 100%.[27] If osteomyelitis is present, the surgical technique can be modified as mentioned, with an additional initial stage to address the infection. The use of an external fixator is indicated during acute infection, and is ideal to stabilize the foot after debridement of infected tissue.[23] Local antibiotic delivery systems are a useful adjunct in these cases as well. The 2 main classes of antibiotic delivery systems are nonbiodegradable systems, such as polymethylmethacrylate beads, and biodegradable systems, such as calcium sulfate/phosphate.[29,30] Although the main disadvantage cited for use of nonbiodegradable systems is the need for additional surgery, it is our preference to use nonbiodegradable systems in these cases because we already plan to return to the operating room for the next stage in the surgical reconstruction. The antibiotics used in these local delivery systems are typically aminoglycosides, which provide good coverage for the most commonly described microbes to cause bone infection, especially chronic osteomyelitis, namely, *Staphylococcus aureus*, Group A beta hemolytic *Streptococcus*, *Enterobacteriaceae*, and *Pseudomonas aeruginosa*.[30] The duration of in vitro elution varies based on the aminoglycoside used, varying from 12 to 220 days, with the peak elution occurring on the first day.[30]

SUMMARY

The LAB technique is an effective tool to add to the surgeon's armamentarium in addressing midfoot Charcot deformities to restore function and decrease the risk of amputation secondary to ulceration and infection. Although this is not the only technique available to address midfoot Charcot, it is an excellent option in cases with significant angular deformity or subluxation, need to reduce shortening of the foot, and in the presence of soft tissue defects, with or without concurrent soft tissue or bone infection.

REFERENCES

1. Center for Disease Control/National Center for Chronic Disease Prevention and Health Promotion. National diabetes statistic report: estimates of diabetes and its burdens in the United States. Atlanta (GA). 2017. Available at: https://www.cdc.gov/diabetes/pdfs/data/statistics/national-diabetes-statistics-report.pdf. Accessed February 1, 2018.
2. Jeffcoate W, Lima J, Nobrega L. The Charcot foot. Diabet Med 2000;17:253–8.
3. Sanders L, Frykberg RG. Diabetic neuropathic osteoarthropathy: the Charcot foot. The high risk foot in diabetes mellitus. New York: Churchill Livingstone; 1991. p. 297–338.
4. Brodsky JW, Rouse AM. Exostectomy for symptomatic bony prominences in diabetic Charcot feet. Clin Orthop Relat Res 1993;296:21–6.
5. Schon LC, Easley ME, Weinfeld SB. Charcot neuroarthropathy of the foot and ankle. Clin Orthop Relat Res 1998;349:116–31.
6. Laborde JM, Philbin TM, Chandler PJ, et al. Preliminary results of primary gastrocnemius-soleus recession for midfoot Charcot arthropathy. Foot Ankle Spec 2016;9(2):140–4.
7. Couppé C, Svensson RB, Kongsgaard M, et al. Human Achilles tendon glycation and function in diabetes. J Appl Physiol (1985) 2016;120:130–7.
8. Lamm BM, Gottlieb HD, Paley D. A two-stage percutaneous approach to Charcot diabetic foot reconstruction. J Foot Ankle Surg 2010;49:517–22.
9. Sohn M, Stuck RM, Pinzur M, et al. Lower-extremity amputation risk after Charcot arthropathy and diabetic foot ulcer. Diabetes Care 2010;33(1):98–100.
10. Smith WB, Moore CA. A proposed treatment algorithm for midfoot Charcot arthropathy. Foot Ankle Spec 2012;5(1):80–4.
11. Bevilacqua NJ, Rogers LC. Surgical management of Charcot midfoot deformities. Clin Podiatr Med Surg 2008;25:81–94.
12. Schweinberger MH, Roukis TS. Surgical correction of soft-tissue ankle equinus contracture. Clin Podiatr Med Surg 2008;25(4):571–85.
13. Conway JD. Charcot salvage of the foot and ankle using external fixation. Foot Ankle Clin N Am 2008;13:157–73.
14. Roukis TS, Zgonis T. Management of acute Charcot fracture-dislocations with the Taylor's Spatial external fixation system. Clin Podiatr Med Surg 2006;23:467–83.
15. Taylor JC. Six-axis deformity analysis and correction. In: Paley D, editor. Principles of deformity correction. Berlin (Germany): Springer-Verlag; 2002. p. 411–36.
16. Siddiqui NA, Pless A. Midfoot and hindfoot Charcot joint deformity correction with hexapod-assisted circular external fixation. Clin Surg 2017;2:1–6.

17. Short DJ, Zgonis T. Management of osteomyelitis and bone loss in the diabetic Charcot foot and ankle. Clin Podiatr Med Surg 2017;34(3):381–7.
18. Sammarco VJ. Superconstructs in Charcot foot deformity. Foot Ankle Clin N Am 2009;14:393–407.
19. Crim BE, Lowery NJ, Wukich DK. Internal fixation techniques for midfoot Charcot neuroarthropathy in patients with diabetes. Clin Podiatr Med Surg 2011;28(4): 673–85.
20. Lamm BM, Siddiqui NA, Nair AK, et al. Intramedullary foot fixation for midfoot Charcot neuroarthropathy. J Foot Ankle Surg 2012;51(4):531–6.
21. Pope EJ, Takemoto RC, Kummer FJ, et al. Midfoot fusion: a biomechanical comparison of plantar plating vs intramedullary screws. Foot Ankle Int 2013;34(3): 409–13.
22. LaFontaine J, Shibuya N, Sampson HW, et al. Trabecular quality and cellular characteristics of normal, diabetic, and Charcot bone. J Foot Ankle Surg 2011;50(6): 648–53.
23. Stapleton JJ, Zgonis T. Surgical reconstruction of the diabetic Charcot foot: internal, external, or combined fixation? Clin Podiatr Med Surg 2012;29(3):425–33.
24. Cullen BD, Weinraub GM, Van Gompel G. Early results with use of the midfoot fusion bolt in Charcot neuroarthropathy. J Foot Ankle Surg 2013;52:235–8.
25. Sammarco VJ, Sammarco GJ, Walker EW Jr, et al. Midtarsal arthrodesis in the treatment of Charcot midfoot arthropathy. J Bone Joint Surg Am 2009;91:80–91.
26. Wiewiorski M, Yasui T, Miska M, et al. Solid bolt fixation of the medial column in Charcot midfoot arthropathy. J Foot Ankle Surg 2013;52(1):88–94.
27. Loredo R, Rahal A, Garcia G, et al. Imaging of the diabetic foot: diagnostic dilemmas. Foot Ankle Spec 2010;3(5):249–64.
28. Palestro CJ, Love C, Tronco GG, et al. Combined labeled leukocyte and technetium 99m sulfur colloid bone marrow imaging for diagnosis musculoskeletal infection. Radiographics 2006;26(3):859–70.
29. Panagopoulous P, Drosos G, Maltezos E, et al. Local antibiotic delivery systems in diabetic foot osteomyelitis: time for one step beyond? Int J Low Extrem Wounds 2015;14(1):87–91.
30. Tsourvakas S. Local antibiotic therapy in the treatment of bone and soft tissue infections. In: Danilla S, editor. Selected topics in reconstructive plastic surgery. Rijeka (Croatia): InTech Europe; 2012. p. 17–44.

Midfoot Charcot Reconstruction

Noman A. Siddiqui, DPM, MHA[a],*, Guido A. LaPorta, DPM, MS[b,c]

KEYWORDS

- Charcot joint • Midfoot Charcot • Bayonet • Intramedullary foot fixation
- Diabetic complications • Neuropathy

KEY POINTS

- Charcot joint should be identified based on stage and location.
- The conservative goal is to prevent significant bony collapse; bony collapse with instability leads to soft tissue complications, which can result in amputation.
- Surgical intervention is often necessary when instability between the forefoot, midfoot, and hindfoot elements exist.
- Medial and lateral column stability play a large role in providing guidance to the degree of surgical intervention required.
- Surgical principles should focus on respecting the soft tissues, obtaining and maintaining correction, and using orthobiologics for improved healing.

INTRODUCTION

Charcot neuroarthropathy can result in a disabling condition that can affect the bones and joints of the foot.[1] Charcot foot most commonly results from peripheral neuropathy leading to loss of protective sensation, autonomic dysfunction, and increased blood flow to the foot. Even though the diabetic foot is the most common cause of Charcot neuroarthropathy, multiple other conditions have also been implicated in creating Charcot joints.[2,3]

Progression of a Charcot joint leads to bone loss and joint subluxations/dislocations, which can distort the normal architecture of the foot and ankle. Long-standing dislocation can result in soft tissue breakdown and arthritis to the neighboring joints.[4,5] Therefore, the normal gait pattern is disrupted making it difficult to ambulate without the assistance of bracing or shoe modifications.[6,7]

Various surgical methods have been described for management of Charcot collapse.[8–11] However, the authors believe that when approaching Charcot foot

Disclosure Statement: None.
a International Center for Limb Lengthening, Rubin Institute for Advanced Orthopedics, Sinai Hospital of Baltimore, 2401 West Belvedere Avenue, Baltimore, MD 21215, USA; b Geisinger CMC, 1800 Mulberry St, Scranton, PA 18510, USA; c Our Lady of Lourdes Memorial Hospital, 169 Riverside Dr, Binghamton, NY 13905, USA
* Corresponding author.
E-mail address: nsiddiqu@lifebridgehealth.org

Clin Podiatr Med Surg 35 (2018) 509–520
https://doi.org/10.1016/j.cpm.2018.07.003
0891-8422/18/© 2018 Elsevier Inc. All rights reserved.

deformity, there are basic deformity planning and management principles that should be considered for conservative or operative treatment. These deformity planning and management principles are presented based on the authors' extensive experience with midfoot Charcot foot deformity correction.

DEFORMITY PLANNING/PREOPERATIVE EVALUATION

Identifying the stage (Eichenholtz classification)[12] and location of the deformity is a simple, primary principle that should be applied whenever managing Charcot joints. Eichenholtz[12] described three stages of Charcot foot that were based on pathologic findings. They are categorized as

I. Development phase
II. Coalescence phase
III. Healing phase

Shibata and colleagues[13] added an additional phase (stage 0), which precedes the developmental phase and during this phase radiographic findings are negative. The mainstays of treatment in the predevelopment and developmental phase are offloading of the affected extremity. During this phase, it is important to rule out any infective process that could have resulted from a previous ulceration or a past history of chronic osteomyelitis. Once the stage has been determined, it is important to note the location of the Charcot deformity. Various authors have classified the Charcot foot based on the anatomic involvement of bones and joints.[2,14,15]

These classifications are useful in communicating the level of Charcot; however, none have been validated as predictive of outcome. The authors believe that location still has a significant role in determination of the type and success of treatment of the Charcot foot deformity.

In the clinical examination, the patient's foot is assessed for areas of ulcerations or preulcerative lesions. These may coincide with bony prominences or locations of instability, thus leading to increased pressure, and must be noted. Evaluating stability in the forefoot, midfoot, and hindfoot can provide insight as to the urgency for operative treatment. A complete vascular examination with particular attention to capillary refill and palpable pulses is noted. The authors recommend a vascular work-up with a vascular surgeon during conservative and/or surgical management of the patient. The foot is also assessed for stability of the bony architecture and equinus deformity. Unstable lateral column Charcot joints result in plantar-central ulcerations of the midfoot and can lead to infection of the midfoot and require surgical intervention to obtain stability. Unstable midfoot Charcot can result in loss of bony and ligamentous stability and dorsiflexion the midfoot onto the hindfoot (ie, "bayonet" effect) (**Fig. 1**). The biomechanical and clinical consequences of bayoneting are discussed in greater detail later in this article. It is important to stabilize the hindfoot and the midfoot when assessing maximum dorsiflexion for presence of equinus. An unstable foot gives the impression of increased dorsiflexion through the midfoot when the Silfverskiöld test is performed.

INDICATIONS FOR SURGERY ON CHARCOT FOOT DEFORMITY

Operating on midfoot Charcot neuropathy is difficult because the risk of complications is higher than in patients without neuropathy. Therefore, clear indications are essential to the success of surgery:

1. Unstable joints/deformity
2. Nonhealing/infected ulcer and/or osteomyelitis

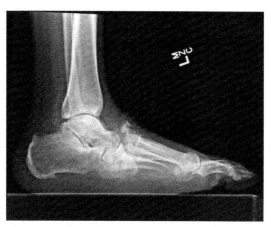

Fig. 1. Lateral view demonstrating collapsing medial arch and "bayonetting" deformity of the forefoot/midfoot on the hindfoot. (Copyright 2018, Rubin Institute for Advanced Orthopedics, Sinai Hospital of Baltimore, Baltimore, MD.)

3. Equinus
4. Deformity is unable to be braced

Surgical Principles

Surgical management of midfoot Charcot deformity should be based on sound surgical principles. Patients with diabetes are known to have poorer healing potential because of advanced glycosylated end products[16] and other comorbidities that can complicate bony and soft tissue healing. Therefore, surgical intervention must take into account all aspects of healing soft tissue and bony elements that are involved in repair.

Respect the soft tissue

Respecting the soft tissue before, during, and after treatment is critical to limiting post-surgical complications. Infections are more common postoperatively in the diabetic population.[17] During stage II or III of a Charcot joint, enough soft tissue edema and erythema has resolved and the clinician can assess the foot and ankle to determine a surgical plan. Taking note of any superficial or deep ulcerations and associated bony prominences assists the surgeon in determining a conservative and/or surgical plan. The overall health of the soft tissue envelope of the foot is important and is affected by chronic edema, prior surgery, and/or trophic changes caused by autonomic neuropathy. Depending on the degree and location of involvement, the surgeon can plan an appropriate surgical approach for correction or offloading techniques to accommodate the deformity. The goal is to maintain a closed skin envelope and prevent ulcerations, which are the precursor of deep infections.

Obtain and maintain correction

In managing Charcot foot, an important principle is to obtain correction and then maintain correction. Conservative measures include such options as total-contact casting, diabetic shoes, and crow walkers. However, if the surgeon determines that conservative measures are not able to protect the patient from violation of principle number one (protect the soft tissue), then the surgeon must use appropriate surgery to correct the deformity.

With this principle, the surgeon must determine the method of correction, which is acute or gradual. In the acute approach, the surgeon accomplishes the goal of obtaining realignment by decreasing the cubic content of bone in the midfoot. Wedge resections are a powerful method and allow for acute realignment. Fixation methods are per the surgeon's preference. However, locked plantar/medial plating and large-diameter axial screw fixation have been reported as successful methods with this technique for correction.[11,18,19]

Gradual correction follows a two-stage method and has been advocated to allow the patient to maintain foot length and to obtain more accurate realignment of the deformed segments.[20] This method combines the use of hexapod external fixation followed by fusion of joints with internal fixation to maintain the correction.[21] Regardless of the method of fixation, the correction is maintained by trying to achieve bony union or fusion.[11,21] When correcting the medial or lateral column, it is vital that surgeons prepare joints to fuse joints. This basic fusion principle is critical to provide stability to the hardware or bony segments. Placing fixation across joints without preparing articular surfaces decreases the likelihood of achieving fusion/union beyond the zone of midfoot collapse.

Orthobiologic supplementation

Autografts have been considered the standard for grafting and supplementation in many aspects of orthopedic and foot and ankle surgery. However, donor site morbidity and quantity of graft have led to the use of allograft material. Allografts have served as an acceptable alternative for structural and inductive scaffold for supplementation.[22] However, in specific populations, such as patients with diabetes, there is evidence that bone biology is affected at the cellular level.[23,24] This can decrease the quality of bone available for fusion.

Advancements in orthobiologics has allowed for the development of various products, such as recombinant human bone morphogenetic protein (rhBMP), platelet-rich plasma, and bone marrow aspirate. Fourman and colleagues[25] performed a retrospective comparative study in 2014 on 82 patients undergoing ankle arthrodesis with external fixation with rhBMP-2. Forty patients did not receive rhBMP-2, and 42 patients received intraoperative rhBMP-2. There were no significant differences in patient demographics, body mass index, diabetes, Charcot joints, tobacco use, and history of infection between the two groups. The results demonstrated 93% union for those receiving rhBMP-2 versus 53% union in the ones who did not receive rhBMP-2. This was verified by computed tomography, which was statistically significant. Additionally, patients treated with rhBMP-2 spent less time in the external fixation than the control (approximately 37 days). Bibbo and colleagues[26] performed a prospective study that looked at the effects of platelet-rich plasma in foot and ankle surgery for 62 high-risk patients. The study found high fusion rates (>90%) of the ankle and hindfoot with the use of platelet-rich plasma. Given that patients with Charcot joints are high risk for nonhealing, it is helpful to supplement the operative site with biologic adjuncts that enhance the environment for the bone to achieve fusion or healing.

EVALUATING THE DEFORMITY

When addressing the patient with midfoot Charcot, the location of the Charcot collapse is identified. After determining this, the surgeon should note whether or not there is an ulceration present. Ulcerations over bony prominences should be approached with suspicion for osteomyelitis. Appropriate diagnostic testing with radiographs, MRI, or nuclear imaging should be used if a bone infection is suspected.

Finally, based on these findings, the surgeon can address the Charcot foot with surgical correction.

Patients with midfoot Charcot can present with or without ulcers. Those without ulcers tend to have collapse on the medial column and may present with varying degrees of stable Lisfranc Charcot. These deformities are seen in patients with Schon type 1A Charcot distribution, which tend disrupt the first and second metatarsals and their respective articulation. These deformities respond well to offloading of bony prominences and conservative management. The key in these deformities is to allow for bony consolidation of the dislocation and to evaluate the patient for equinus deformity via the Silfverskiöld test.

Those who do not have an equinus contracture tend to do better than those who have an equinus contracture. Patients who have equinus tend to develop ulcers over bony prominences. In those instances, surgical intervention can focus on bony prominence resection and a tendo-Achilles lengthening. At our facility, we tend to perform a gastroc-soleus recession along with bony protuberance exostectomy. The gastroc-soleus recession is preferred over the Hoke triple-hemisection because it is better at maintaining push-off strength and decreases the risk of a calcaneus gait, which is a complication of the latter.

Midfoot Charcot deformities with ulcers become more common because the Charcot deformity progresses more proximal as seen in Schon type 2 and 3. In these types of patients, it is important to note if the ulcer is medial or lateral. Lateral ulcers are a sign of greater instability and a disruption of the lateral column, and the patient is on a path to the classic "rockerbottom" deformity. This collapse is exacerbated by the effect of the ground reaction vector that is initiated at heel strike (**Fig. 2**). This repetitive act only assists in further dislocation of the lateral column. In this population, an equinus contracture further exacerbates this lateral column disruption and many patients develop an ulceration of the plantar lateral foot. The ulceration is maintained by the "bayoneting" effect of the forefoot on the hindfoot, which is commonly seen in these types of deformities (see **Fig. 1**). Medial ulcers occur when there is peritalar dislocation of the navicular-cuneiform joint and the talus dislocates medial and plantar. The authors believe that these deformities must be addressed surgically to create a stable foot and ankle complex. Correction is performed acutely via wedge resections or gradually using hexapod devices. If there is a history of ulceration or osteomyelitis, the authors always stage the correction to minimize the risk of future infection. When undertaking a midfoot Charcot reconstruction, the authors aim is to accomplish the following:

- Maintain anatomic realignment
- Use minimally invasive fixation technique
- Obtain formal multiple joint fusion
- Achieve joint fixation/fusion beyond the level of Charcot collapse
- Select rigid fixation
- Preserve foot length
- Combine with external fixation if necessary

This is accomplished in various methods; however, the authors prefer to use the intramedullary foot fixation technique with some modifications as described next.[21]

SURGICAL TECHNIQUE

The authors use a percutaneous technique to ensure the proper placement of intramedullary foot fixation. The patient is supine on a radiolucent table with a bump under the

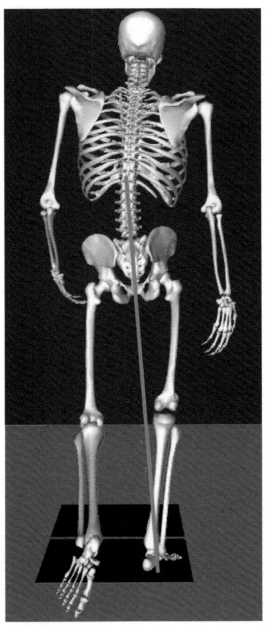

Fig. 2. Ground reaction force vector starts at the level of the calcaneocuboid joint laterally to the level of T10. (Copyright 2018, Rubin Institute for Advanced Orthopedics, Sinai Hospital of Baltimore, Baltimore, MD.)

ipsilateral hip to obtain a foot-forward position. A thigh tourniquet is applied to the lower extremity. The extremity is prepared in an aseptic fashion to the level of the tourniquet, providing the ability to flex the knee during the procedure. A gastroc-soleus recession is performed to resolve any equinus contracture. A limited open technique for preparation is performed on joints that will be fixated along the medial and lateral column. Temporary fixation with smooth wires to obtain alignment is performed. Then a 1.8-mm Ilizarov wire is inserted from the plantar aspect of the first metatarsophalangeal joint to the center of the first metatarsal head by maximum dorsiflexion of the first metatarsophalangeal joint (**Fig. 3**). A lateral fluoroscopic view ensures that the direction of the wire is parallel and coincides with the lateral anatomic axis of the first metatarsal (see **Fig. 3**). The guide pin is advanced manually with a mallet to the level of the base of the first metatarsal, which ensures intramedullary placement of the guide pin. The goal of lateral column stabilization is to obtain a formal fusion of the calcaneocuboid joint. A 1.8-mm Ilizarov wire is inserted through the interosseous structures of the third and fourth intermetatarsal bases. A stab incision is made dorsally at the insertion site of the 1.8-mm wire. Blunt dissection is carried down to the metatarsal base. A 4.8-mm cannulated drill bit is then inserted over the 1.8-mm wire and then drilled into the anterior portions of the calcaneus. The drill, along with the 1.8-mm wire, are removed and replaced with the guide pin from the 6.5/7.0/8.0-mm cannulated screw set. After confirmation of proper insertion on the anteroposterior and lateral fluoroscopic views, the three screws are inserted.

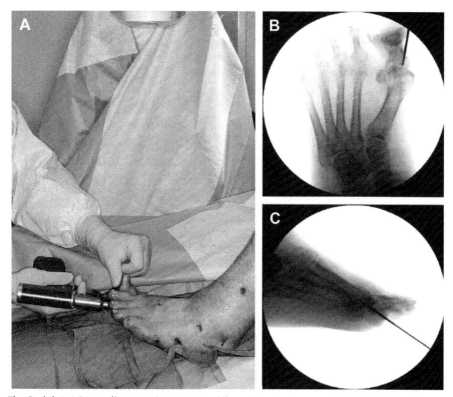

Fig. 3. (*A*) A 1.8-mm Ilizarov wire is inserted from the plantar aspect of the first metatarsophalangeal joint to the center of the first metatarsal head by maximum dorsiflexion of the first metatarsophalangeal joint. (*B*) The 1.8-mm Ilizarov wire is placed on the equator of the metatarsal head. (*C*) Lateral fluoroscopic view ensures that the direction of the wire is parallel and coincides with the lateral anatomic axis of the first metatarsal. (Copyright 2018, Rubin Institute for Advanced Orthopedics, Sinai Hospital of Baltimore, Baltimore, MD.)

The head of the screws are buried into the bone. Compression occurs once the screw engages the talar and calcaneal body. However, the authors focus is to provide stability and it is not imperative to achieve compression along the medial and lateral columns.

The authors have incorporated subtalar joint fusions as a part of the final construct to impart hindfoot stability to the medial and lateral columns in Charcot joints. A standard medial approach is used to prepare the articular surfaces of the subtalar joint and fully threaded 6.5/7.0/8.0-mm fixation is used to achieve compression across the hindfoot.

The plantar incisions are then closed with 3.0 Monocryl sutures (Ethicon Inc, Somerville, NJ). The patient is placed in a 90° bivalved non–weightbearing short leg cast for the initial postoperative course. The patient is seen 1 week postoperatively, and skin incisions are evaluated. The patient is then placed in a non–weightbearing short-leg cast for a total of 8 weeks, with intermittent follow-up. External fixation is used to protect and offload internal fixation. It is a useful adjunct for these procedures to allow earlier load transfer for this patient population who may have difficulty with prolonged cast immobilization.

The authors address the equinus component that tends to reoccur months after reconstructive surgery. We routinely check for recurrent equinus and believe if there is no residual equinus component, there is less likelihood of collapse that results in ulceration in the future. In the authors experience, even if midfoot collapse reoccurs (because of broken hardware, partial/incomplete fusion, pseudoarthrosis), as long as the foot functions as a solid unit and has adequate ankle dorsiflexion, then the patient's chances for recurrent ulceration decreases.

CASE EXAMPLE
Midfoot Charcot Correction with Internal and External Fixation

A 72-year-old African American man presented with midfoot Charcot deformity of the left foot. He had received treatment from other physicians for many weeks for chronic gout, cellulitis, and an "ankle sprain." Patient related no prior trauma or history of gout before this episode. A referral to the author was prompted when persistent pedal edema and signs of a preulcerative lesion were noted with no skin breakdown. Patient denied any pain to the left foot and had been ambulating in left CAM boot walker, as recommended by another physician. He was in excellent medical health but related a well-controlled past medical history of diabetes mellitus type II, hypertension, and hyperlipidemia.

Clinically, he presented with an edematous foot with no erythema or signs of acute infection. The soft tissue envelope was intact; however, a sign of a preulcerative lesion was noted plantar centrally in the midfoot. Excellent pulses, capillary refill, and normal temperature gradient was appreciated. Loss of protective sensation was noted with Semmes-Weinstein monofilament examination. He had supple range of motion in the hindfoot but gross instability was noted of the medial and lateral columns of the midfoot and forefoot. His radiographic evaluation indicated midfoot Lisfranc/perinavicular Charcot joints with bone loss and comminution. A collapsed Meary angle and bayonetting of the forefoot to hindfoot were observed (see **Fig. 1**). Combining the clinical and radiographic findings allowed the foot to be classified as Eichenholtz stage 2 with radiographic characteristics of a Schon 3/4 deformity. Formal vascular studies were conducted, which were positive for excellent perfusion to the extremity. The patient consented to surgical intervention.

A two-stage correction was used that obtained gradual distraction and realignment of the midfoot deformity with hexapod external fixation (**Fig. 4**). Once the correction was achieved, the realignment was maintained with focused joint fusions (as described previously) and placement of internal and external fixation (**Fig. 5**). The external fixation device was used to protect the internal construct during the healing phase and a load-sharing device for the patient's activities of daily living. The sutures were removed at 3 weeks, and he was allowed to shower and to ambulate for most activities with the assistance of a walker. He had an overall uneventful postoperative course. If there was a concern for a pin-related infection, it was managed immediately with orally administered antibiotics. Approximately 10 weeks after surgery, the external fixation device was removed when radiographic signs of bony consolidation were observed. After frame removal, the foot

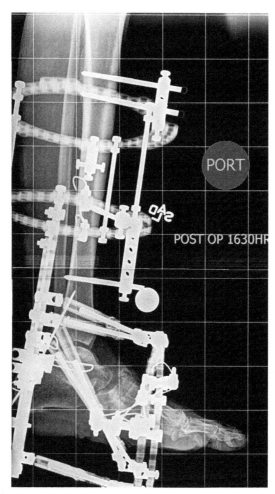

Fig. 4. Stage 1 of the correction involved application of multiplanar hexapod external fixation to obtain gradual correction of the deformity. The hindfoot was acutely corrected with tendo-Achilles lengthening and extra-articular pinning of the ankle joint. (Copyright 2018, Rubin Institute for Advanced Orthopedics, Sinai Hospital of Baltimore, Baltimore, MD.)

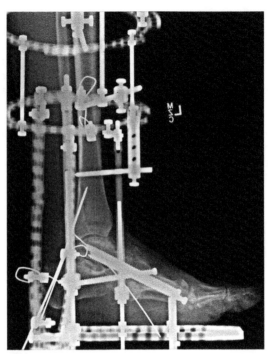

Fig. 5. Stage 2 of the correction (after gradual correction) involved formal fusion of all medial and lateral column joints with internal fixation using the intramedullary foot fixation technique. (Copyright 2018, Rubin Institute for Advanced Orthopedics, Sinai Hospital of Baltimore, Baltimore, MD.)

was protected in a short CAM walker boot for 8 months. The boot was converted to an Arizona brace with protective extra depth diabetic footwear. The patient had a positive outcome that has been maintained for many years after the reconstruction (**Fig. 6**).

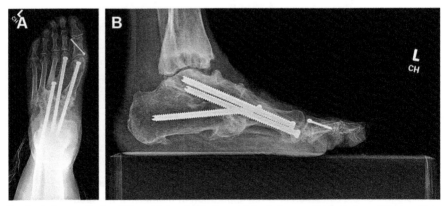

Fig. 6. Anteroposterior (*A*) and lateral (*B*) views of foot show solid fusion and that realignment was maintained of the medial and lateral columns. (Copyright 2018, Rubin Institute for Advanced Orthopedics, Sinai Hospital of Baltimore, Baltimore, MD.)

SUMMARY

Midfoot Charcot deformity is one of the more complex pathologies encountered by foot and ankle surgeons. Nonoperative treatment with total contact casting, immobilization, and use of an AFO, such as a Charcot restraint orthotic walker, are reliable methods to treat this complex condition. However, in cases that involve unstable joints/deformity, nonhealing foot ulcers with or without osteomyelitis, equinus, and a nonbraceable-deformity, often it becomes necessary to intervene with operative methods to salvage a limb. There are many methods to address the condition, and the authors have demonstrated methods to correct the deformity successfully. However, the authors believe that it is more important to focus on surgical principles and rely on hardware and biologic products as adjuncts to support the principles of correction that are described.

REFERENCES

1. Williams RH, Larsen PR. Complications of diabetes mellitus: the diabetic foot. Williams textbook of endocrinology. 12th edition. Philadelphia: Saunders; 2003.
2. Sanders LJ, Frykberg RG. The Charcot foot. In: Bowker JH, Pfeifer MA, editors. Levin and O'Neal's the diabetic foot. 7th edition. Philadelphia: Mosby/Elsevier; 2008. p. 257–83.
3. Frykberg RG, Belczyk R. Epidemiology of the Charcot foot. Clin Podiatr Med Surg 2008;25(1):17–28, v.
4. Lamm BM. Surgical reconstruction and stepwise approach to acute Charcot neuroarthropathy. In: Thomas Zgonis T, editor. Surgical reconstruction of the diabetic foot and ankle. Philadelphia: Lippincott Williams & Wilkins; 2009. p. 223–9.
5. Zonno AJ, Myerson MS. Surgical correction of midfoot arthritis with and without deformity. Foot Ankle Clin 2011;16(1):35–47.
6. Sinacore DR, Mueller MJ. Off-loading for diabetic foot disease. In: Levin ME, O'Neal LW, Bowker JH, et al, editors. Levin and O'Neal's the diabetic foot. Philadelphia: Mosby/Elsevier; 2008. p. 287–303.
7. Armin K. Rehabilitation and therapeutic footwear for the reconstructed and amputee patient. In: Zgonis T, editor. Surgical reconstruction of the diabetic foot and ankle. Philadelphia: Lippincott Williams & Wilkins; 2009. p. 411–25.
8. Bevilacqua NJ, Rogers LC. Surgical management of Charcot midfoot deformities. Clin Podiatr Med Surg 2008;25(1):81–94, vii.
9. Pinzur MS. The role of ring external fixation in Charcot foot arthropathy. Foot Ankle Clin 2006;11(4):837–47.
10. Lamm BM, Gottlieb HD, Paley D. A two-stage percutaneous approach to Charcot diabetic foot reconstruction. J Foot Ankle Surg 2010;49(6):517–22.
11. Sammarco VJ. Superconstructs in the treatment of Charcot foot deformity: plantar plating, locked plating, and axial screw fixation. Foot Ankle Clin 2009;14(3): 393–407.
12. Eichenholtz SN. Charcot joints. Springfield (IL): Charles C. Thomas; 1966.
13. Shibata T, Tada K, Hashizume C. The results of arthrodesis of the ankle for leprotic neuroarthropathy. J Bone Joint Surg 1990;72A:749–56.
14. Brodsky JW, Rouse AM. Exostectomy for symptomatic bony prominences in diabetic Charcot feet. Clin Orthop Relat Res 1993;296:21–6.
15. Schon LC, Weinfeld SB, Horton GA, et al. Radiographic and clinical classification of acquired midtarsus deformities. Foot Ankle Int 1998;19(6):394–404.
16. Ahmed N. Advanced glycation endproducts: role in pathology of diabetic complications. Diabetes Res Clin Pract 2005;67(1):3–21.

17. Stryker LS, Abdel MP, Morrey ME, et al. Elevated postoperative blood glucose and preoperative hemoglobin A1C are associated with increased wound complications following total joint arthroplasty. J Bone Joint Surg Am 2013;95(9):808–14. S1–2.

18. Grant WP, Garcia-Lavin S, Sabo R. Beaming the columns for Charcot diabetic foot reconstruction: a retrospective analysis. J Foot Ankle Surg 2011;50(2):182–9.

19. Nasser EM, LaPorta GA, Trott K. Medial column arthrodesis using an anatomic distal fibular locking plate. J Foot Ankle Surg 2015;54(4):671–6.

20. Siddiqui NA, Pless A. Midfoot and hindfoot Charcot joint deformity correction with hexapod-assisted circular external fixation. Clin Surg 2017;2:1430.

21. Lamm BM, Siddiqui NA, Nair AK, et al. Intramedullary foot fixation for midfoot Charcot neuroarthropathy. J Foot Ankle Surg 2012;51(4):531–6.

22. Malinin TI, Carpenter EM, Temple HT. Particulate bone allograft incorporation in regeneration of osseous defects; importance of particle sizes. Open Orthop J 2007;1:19–24.

23. La Fontaine J, Shibuya N, Sampson HW, et al. Trabecular quality and cellular characteristics of normal, diabetic, and Charcot bone. J Foot Ankle Surg 2011;50(6):648–53.

24. Saito M, Fujii K, Mori Y, et al. Role of collagen enzymatic and glycation induced cross-links as a determinant of bone quality in spontaneously diabetic WBN/Kob rats. Osteoporos Int 2006;17(10):1514–23.

25. Fourman MS, Borst EW, Bogner E, et al. Recombinant human BMP-2 increases the incidence and rate of healing in complex ankle arthrodesis. Clin Orthop Relat Res 2014;472(2):732–9.

26. Bibbo C, Bono CM, Lin SS. Union rates using autologous platelet concentrate alone and with bone graft in high-risk foot and ankle surgery patients. J Surg Orthop Adv 2005;14(1):17–22.

UNITED STATES POSTAL SERVICE ®

Statement of Ownership, Management, and Circulation
(All Periodicals Publications Except Requester Publications)

1. Publication Title	2. Publication Number	3. Filing Date
CLINICS IN PODIATRIC MEDICINE & SURGERY	000 – 707	9/18/2018

4. Issue Frequency	5. Number of Issues Published Annually	6. Annual Subscription Price
JAN, APR, JUL, OCT	4	$294.00

7. Complete Mailing Address of Known Office of Publication (Not printer) (Street, city, county, state, and ZIP+4®)

ELSEVIER INC.
230 Park Avenue, Suite 800
New York, NY 10169

Contact Person
STEPHEN R. BUSHING
Telephone (Include area code)
215-239-3688

8. Complete Mailing Address of Headquarters or General Business Office of Publisher (Not printer)

ELSEVIER INC.
230 Park Avenue, Suite 800
New York, NY 10169

9. Full Names and Complete Mailing Addresses of Publisher, Editor, and Managing Editor (Do not leave blank)

Publisher (Name and complete mailing address)

TAYLOR E BALL, ELSEVIER INC.
1600 JOHN F KENNEDY BLVD. SUITE 1800
PHILADELPHIA, PA 19103-2899

Editor (Name and complete mailing address)

LAUREN BOYLE, ELSEVIER INC.
1600 JOHN F KENNEDY BLVD. SUITE 1800
PHILADELPHIA, PA 19103-2899

Managing Editor (Name and complete mailing address)

PATRICK MANLEY, ELSEVIER INC.
1600 JOHN F KENNEDY BLVD. SUITE 1800
PHILADELPHIA, PA 19103-2899

10. Owner (Do not leave blank. If the publication is owned by a corporation, give the name and address of the corporation immediately followed by the names and addresses of all stockholders owning or holding 1 percent or more of the total amount of stock. If not owned by a corporation, give the names and addresses of the individual owners. If owned by a partnership or other unincorporated firm, give its name and address as well as those of each individual owner. If the publication is published by a nonprofit organization, give its name and address.)

Full Name	Complete Mailing Address
WHOLLY OWNED SUBSIDIARY OF REED/ELSEVIER, US HOLDINGS	1600 JOHN F KENNEDY BLVD. SUITE 1800 PHILADELPHIA, PA 19103-2899

11. Known Bondholders, Mortgagees, and Other Security Holders Owning or Holding 1 Percent or More of Total Amount of Bonds, Mortgages, or Other Securities. If none, check box ► ☐ None

Full Name	Complete Mailing Address
N/A	

12. Tax Status (For completion by nonprofit organizations authorized to mail at nonprofit rates) (Check one)
The purpose, function, and nonprofit status of this organization and the exempt status for federal income tax purposes:
☒ Has Not Changed During Preceding 12 Months
☐ Has Changed During Preceding 12 Months (Publisher must submit explanation of change with this statement)

PS Form **3526**, July 2014 [Page 1 of 4 (see instructions page 4)] PSN: 7530-01-000-9931 PRIVACY NOTICE: See our privacy policy on www.usps.com

---

13. Publication Title			14. Issue Date for Circulation Data Below	
CLINICS IN PODIATRIC MEDICINE & SURGERY			JULY 2018	

15. Extent and Nature of Circulation			Average No. Copies Each Issue During Preceding 12 Months	No. Copies of Single Issue Published Nearest to Filing Date
a. Total Number of Copies (Net press run)			193	249
b. Paid Circulation (By Mail and Outside the Mail)	(1)	Mailed Outside-County Paid Subscriptions Stated on PS Form 3541 (Include paid distribution above nominal rate, advertiser's proof copies, and exchange copies)	117	148
	(2)	Mailed In-County Paid Subscriptions Stated on PS Form 3541 (Include paid distribution above nominal rate, advertiser's proof copies, and exchange copies)	0	0
	(3)	Paid Distribution Outside the Mails Including Sales Through Dealers and Carriers, Street Vendors, Counter Sales, and Other Paid Distribution Outside USPS®	13	17
	(4)	Paid Distribution by Other Classes of Mail Through the USPS (e.g., First-Class Mail®)	0	0
c. Total Paid Distribution (Sum of 15b (1), (2), (3), and (4))		►	130	165
d. Free or Nominal Rate Distribution (By Mail and Outside the Mail)	(1)	Free or Nominal Rate Outside-County Copies included on PS Form 3541	53	69
	(2)	Free or Nominal Rate In-County Copies included on PS Form 3541	0	0
	(3)	Free or Nominal Rate Copies Mailed at Other Classes Through the USPS (e.g., First-Class Mail)	0	0
	(4)	Free or Nominal Rate Distribution Outside the Mail (Carriers or other means)	0	0
e. Total Free or Nominal Rate Distribution (Sum of 15d (1), (2), (3) and (4))		►	53	69
f. Total Distribution (Sum of 15c and 15e)		►	183	234
g. Copies not Distributed (See Instructions to Publishers #4 (page #3))		►	10	15
h. Total (Sum of 15f and g)		►	193	249
i. Percent Paid (15c divided by 15f times 100)			71.04%	70.51%

* If you are claiming electronic copies, go to line 16 on page 3. If you are not claiming electronic copies, skip to line 17 on page 3.

16. Electronic Copy Circulation		Average No. Copies Each Issue During Preceding 12 Months	No. Copies of Single Issue Published Nearest to Filing Date
a. Paid Electronic Copies	►	0	0
b. Total Paid Print Copies (Line 15c) + Paid Electronic Copies (Line 16a)	►	130	165
c. Total Print Distribution (Line 15f) + Paid Electronic Copies (Line 16a)	►	183	234
d. Percent Paid (Both Print & Electronic Copies) (16b divided by 16c × 100)	►	71.04%	70.51%

☒ I certify that 50% of all my distributed copies (electronic and print) are paid above a nominal price.

17. Publication of Statement of Ownership

☒ If the publication is a general publication, publication of this statement is required. Will be printed in the OCTOBER 2018 issue of this publication. ☐ Publication not required.

18. Signature and Title of Editor, Publisher, Business Manager, or Owner

STEPHEN R. BUSHING - INVENTORY DISTRIBUTION CONTROL MANAGER

Stephen R. Bushing Date 9/18/2018

I certify that all information furnished on this form is true and complete. I understand that anyone who furnishes false or misleading information on this form or who omits material or information requested on the form may be subject to criminal sanctions (including fines and imprisonment) and/or civil sanctions (including civil penalties).

PS Form **3526**, July 2014 (Page 3 of 4) PRIVACY NOTICE: See our privacy policy on www.usps.com

Printed and bound by CPI Group (UK) Ltd, Croydon, CR0 4YY

03/10/2024

01040398-0017